OUTCOMES OF COMMUNITY CARE FOR USERS AND CARERS

A SOCIAL SERVICES PERSPECTIVE

OUTCOMES OF COMMUNITY CARE FOR USERS AND CARERS

A SOCIAL SERVICES PERSPECTIVE

Andrew Nocon and Hazel Qureshi

OPEN UNIVERSITY PRESS
Buckingham • Philadelphia

Open University Press
Celtic Court
22 Ballmoor
Buckingham
MK18 1XW

and
1900 Frost Road, Suite 101
Bristol, PA 19007, USA

First Published 1996
Reprinted 1998

A catalogue record of this book is available from the British Library

ISBN 0 335 19668 3 (pb)   0 335 19669 1 (hb)

Library of Congress Cataloging-in-Publication Data
Nocon, Andrew, 1951–
    Outcomes of community care for users and carers : a social
services perspective / Andrew Nocon and Hazel Qureshi.
        p.   cm.
    Includes bibliographical references and index.
    ISBN 0–335–19669–1   ISBN 0–335–19668–3 (pbk.)
    1. Community health services—Evaluation.   2. Social service
—Evaluation.   I. Qureshi, Hazel. II. Title.
RA427.N62 1996
362.1′2—dc20   95–49669
                                                          CIP

Typeset by Graphicraft Typesetters Limited, Hong Kong
Printed in Great Britain by St Edmundsbury Press,
Bury St Edmunds, Suffolk

CONTENTS

ACKNOWLEDGEMENTS

This work was undertaken by the Social Policy Research Unit, University of York, which receives support from the Department of Health; the views expressed in this publication are those of the authors and not necessarily those of the Department of Health. Nevertheless, we should like to thank the Department of Health, and in particular the Research and Development Division, for their funding of the review on which this book is based, and for supporting us in our wish to expand, revise and update it for wider publication in the light of the intense current interest in the subject of outcomes.

In addition, we are very grateful to Catherine Thompson for preparing a first draft of Chapter 5; to Sally Baldwin, Ian Sinclair and the anonymous reviewers for their helpful comments on earlier versions; to Lorna Foster for proofreading and Jenny Bowes for secretarial support and an unfailing ability to decipher and reorganize our numerous revisions; and, not least, to Jacinta Evans of Open University Press for her encouragement, enthusiasm and support.

INTRODUCTION

The need to evaluate the outcomes of social care has long been recognized. Such evaluation provides a means of public accountability, it enables the effectiveness and cost-effectiveness of social care to be measured and it offers a safeguard against the general introduction of new, unproven methods of intervention (Goldberg and Connelly 1982; Cheetham *et al.* 1992). In practice, however, performance measurement has focused on activity indicators, on inputs and processes, rather than on outcomes for service users. Knowing how many hours of home care are being provided to a user does not indicate how effectively that person's needs are being met. Nor do destinational outcomes, such as admissions to residential care, indicate whether such admissions are appropriate for the individual concerned.

The introduction of new community care arrangements in 1993 has made the need for outcome evaluation even more important. These arrangements were intended to address users' and carers' needs more directly and more effectively than under the previous service-led system. Care management involves both the systematic assessment of users' and carers' needs and the purchase of services to meet those needs. While community care plans offer a framework within which objectives can be set, service contracts provide a means to secure services to meet users' and carers' needs. Outcome measures are then needed to monitor how effectively users' and carers' needs are being met and whether services meet the defined objectives (Audit Commission 1992a; Department of Health 1993). While the Social Services Inspectorate (SSI) and NHS Executive report that Social Services Departments generally recognize the need to focus on outcomes, there is little evidence so far of outcome measurement in practice (Department of Health 1994). Some authorities are certainly carrying out satisfaction surveys, but these often focus on users' evaluation of process rather than the specific benefits or impacts of services; as will be discussed, the meaning of 'satisfaction' is often unclear in any case. Nor is the contracting process being used to specify desired outcomes for users and carers – other than perhaps in global terms which would be difficult to monitor.

The lack of evidence of outcome measurement in community care should not be surprising. Community care is a broad and complex concept which may have different meanings for professional staff, managers, users and carers. Research projects which have focused on, for example, the relocation of former long-stay hospital residents into the community have used a daunting array of instruments to examine the many areas of people's lives that might be affected by the provision of community facilities. For people already living in the community, individual services may be designed to have a more specific impact. Nevertheless, the same service can assist people in different ways, and unintended consequences should also be taken into account, whether positive or negative. Outcome measures should be sufficiently flexible and broad ranging to encompass these various possibilities. A further issue concerns attribution. It is difficult enough to determine changes in people's lives. But to state with any certainty that they are due to identified interventions or services requires a proof of causality that may well be elusive: even where correlations can be established, it may be impossible to identify all the extraneous factors that may have some bearing on the outcomes themselves.

This book is in three parts. Part I considers background and contextual issues and Chapter 1 will examine the different ways in which the term 'outcome' has been used. Clarity about its meaning is a prerequisite if the focus of measurement is to be clear. It will also provide a discussion of the policy context within which outcome measurement is to take place. Chapter 2 will consider the opportunities currently available to incorporate outcome measurement into the work and practices of Social Services Departments. The possibilities for such measurement exist in a number of recent developments, including quality initiatives, performance measurement, community care plans, contracting, inspection procedures, assessment and care management. Despite the potential offered by such developments, however, outcome measurement remains underdeveloped.

One of the central features of the community care arrangements is the need to take account of service users' and carers' own definitions of their needs and of the services they require. It follows that the desired outcomes should similarly reflect their views. Chapter 3 will, therefore, examine some of the statements that users and carers have made about their expectations of community care. Their views will provide a benchmark against which outcome measures can be assessed.

A number of such measures will be reviewed in Part II of the book, with individual chapters being devoted to measures for the larger groups of users and for carers. Many of the measures discussed have been developed in a health care context, although there is often an overlap with the needs that social care services seek to address. Other measures will have been used in broader research contexts, perhaps to examine very specific aspects of people's lives.

While the individual chapters in Part II indicate the potential usefulness or weaknesses of existing measures, the conclusions, in Part III, draw together the broader issues arising from this review. One prominent theme which has to be acknowledged is the absence of user or carer input in the development of most existing measures. This should not be taken as an indictment of all current measures. Nevertheless, it does reflect the professional interests that underpin the measures: the principle of user and carer centrality in needs assessment, and consequently in outcome evaluation, requires that any measures designed to examine outcomes should take account of users' and carers' perspectives. Second, the stated policy objectives of the new community care arrangements emphasize the importance of user choice, independence, involvement in decision-making, and control over the nature and process of service provision. Such objectives, too, need to be incorporated into outcome measurement, and systematic means need to be designed to achieve this. Finally, if measurement of outcomes is to become part of everyday practice, then issues of organizational and professional culture will have to be tackled to create a context in which outcome measurement can be valid and practically useful.

Measuring community care outcomes will not be easy: the specific focus of any measures will need to be clarified; the different needs of different user groups and of individual users may need to be addressed in different ways; the operational advantage of brief, simple measures has to be balanced against the limited amount of information they will provide and the practical problems associated with more complex measures; validity and reliability have to be established; and – not least – practitioners have to be convinced of the value of the collection of outcome data in routine practice. The final chapter concludes with some suggestions about the way that such issues might be addressed.

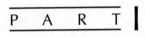

PART I

CONCEPTS AND THEMES

CHAPTER 1

CONCEPTUAL ISSUES AND POLICY CONTEXT

Introduction

This chapter sets the scene for the consideration of outcome measurement in community care. It first aims to clarify the definition of 'outcome' which is used throughout the book, and to examine the use of the term in the literature on social care. This leads to an identification of the questions which need to answered in order to put into place the elements that are needed for outcome measurement. Discussion of the applicability of these elements to community care makes it clear that, although technical and professional knowledge can be useful, the identification and measurement of outcomes cannot be value-free. As Smith (1996) observes, outcome measurement in routine practice is intended as a control mechanism, designed to give feedback to organizations, or individuals, about the effectiveness of services, with an expectation that such information will be interpreted and used as a basis for action. The question of routine measurement therefore has to be considered in context. The chapter concludes with an examination of those features of the service and policy context which have been important in determining a renewed emphasis on the need for an understanding of outcomes for service users and carers.

Conceptual issues

Definition of 'outcome'

An 'outcome' is broadly understood to be the impact, effect or consequence of a service or a policy. In this broad sense, a change in service structure or process may be viewed as the outcome of policy. For example, the introduction of arrangements for assessment and care management within local authorities may be seen as an outcome of current community care policy. This book is not concerned with outcomes of this kind, but rather with impacts on users of services and their carers. The term 'outcome' is often used rather loosely and may have a range of meanings, but consideration of the literature helps to clarify the ways in which a distinction has been drawn between intermediate and final outcomes, and how the relationships between objectives, needs, service inputs and outcomes have been conceptualized.

Concepts and use of terms

Knapp (1984: 22), developing ideas about the economics of social care, conceived the interlinking of objectives, needs and outputs as:

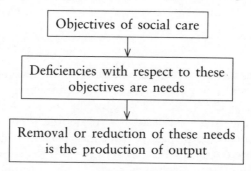

Knapp distinguished between final output, defined as the reduction of welfare shortfall for service users, and intermediate output, defined in terms of receipt of services (ibid.: 22, 32). This work reflected an economic perspective, described as the production of welfare approach, which has been subsequently developed and widely applied, although the term 'outcome' is now used in preference to 'output'. The production of welfare model (Davies and Challis 1986) is a quantitative model which relates final outcomes to measures of both resource and non-resource inputs, the latter including, for example, the characteristics of clients. Proponents of this model have always clearly spelt out that final outputs or outcomes are effects upon the welfare of service users (Challis 1981; Challis and Davies 1986) and should be distinguished from intermediate outcomes which are changes in services. However, as will become evident, the terms 'output', 'outcome', 'intermediate' and 'final' appear in different contexts throughout the literature and their usage is not entirely consistent.

  Cheetham *et al.* (1992) objected to the labels 'intermediate' and 'final', and, implicitly, to the word 'output', on the grounds that these terms reflect economic jargon and are less intuitively clear than their suggested alternative terms: 'service-based outcomes' and 'client-based outcomes'. Cheetham *et al.* pointed out that, for some studies, service-based outcomes may be final outcomes in the sense that changes in service characteristics may be all that is required from a particular policy or all that it is possible to measure. They also emphasized that what one person may see as an input may be seen as an outcome by someone else. For example, an outcome of community care service for a particular client may be access to another service, such as dental care or a medical check for people living in supported accommodation.

Subjective and objective quality of life

Shiell *et al.* (1990) drew a distinction between service characteristics and effects on service users, but suggested reserving the title 'output' for the former and 'outcome' for the latter, because they argued that this made clearer the difference between quality of service and the client's eventual quality of life. The latter, for Shiell *et al.*, was defined in strictly subjective terms – as the extent to which an individual feels his or her needs have been met. In contrast, some commentators would consider a characteristic of a residential setting – such as its 'domestic' appearance – to be an 'objective' measure of quality of life in relation to an individual, and therefore would count this as part of an assessment of final outcome. For others, this would be seen strictly as a measure of service quality, or quality of care, and only as possibly intermediate in producing a final effect on the well-being of a person resident there (Raynes 1986).

Measuring quality of life is often considered to require the investigation of both subjective elements, such as life satisfaction or well-being, and more objective elements reflecting external life conditions (Barry *et al.* 1992; Perry and Felce 1995). Thus, if there was an interest in social contacts, the number and frequency of contacts might be measured as well as the expressed degree of satisfaction with such contacts. Felce and Perry (1995) argue that a person's expressed satisfaction with a particular aspect of their life should not be confused with their estimate of its relative importance to them. Clearly, this is of particular significance if people are only asked for satisfaction ratings in areas which do not matter much to them: a quite misleading picture of quality of life might be given. In general, both objective and subjective aspects should be measured, since there is a balance to be struck between ensuring that individuals receive services which they value, and ensuring a distribution of resources which is seen to be fair in terms of the opportunities offered to people in similar situations (Culyer 1990). Data about so-called objective factors may be collected by a variety of methods, relying either on self-report, perhaps through an interview or diary study, or on observation, or the reports of third parties. Subjective factors seem to require a direct response from the subject, although as will be outlined, the elicitation of evaluative views from some individuals can present considerable difficulties.

All the above definitions are summarized in Box 1.1.

Box 1.1   Outcomes for individuals: summary of terms

Outcome – impact, effect or consequence

Intermediate outcome – receipt of services

Final outcome – effect or impact on service user or carer

Process – way in which services are combined and delivered

Objective – intended aim or goal. Objectives may relate to process or outcomes

Domain – area of a person's life where impact is intended (for example: social integration, emotional well-being)

Subjective aspect of quality of life – expression of a person's evaluative feelings about a domain (for example, satisfaction or importance)

Objective aspect of quality of life – externally observable life condition reflecting a domain (for example: number of social contacts, 'domestic' appearance of environment)

Timescale of effects

In discussing outcome measurement for children, Parker *et al.* (1991) at times used the terms 'intermediate' and 'final' in the same sense as they are used in the production of welfare approach (ibid.: 57) but in other parts of their book use 'intermediate' and 'final' in relation to the timescale along which effects may be expected (ibid.: 24, 29). Thus, taking a view of outcomes as sequences of events, the final outcomes of child care may be observable only in adulthood, and the more immediate impacts of services are only intermediate steps towards these. In the short term, however, it is possible to measure only intermediate outcomes (which in this usage of the term are still impacts on clients, rather than service characteristics). There is, nonetheless, a problem that some short-term effects may disappear after a time, or prove less important in the longer term than might have been supposed. For example, some of the demonstrable short-term effects of early intervention with young disabled children proved, in the longer term, to be short lived (Sloper *et al.* 1986). Equally, unanticipated outcomes may appear in the longer term: a long-running study of families who received early intervention demonstrated an unexpected connection between early intervention and later parental confidence, reflected in, among other things, much higher rates of employment among mothers whose children had received early intervention (Cunningham *et al.* 1986).

The timescale of measurement and the degree to which unanticipated outcomes are detected will continue to present difficulties in the collection and interpretation of outcome data. It can be difficult to define end-points in community care, particularly for groups such as people with learning disability, where the involvement of services may be long term. The outcomes of preventative services are often difficult to demonstrate because of the large number of other factors involved in people's lives in the longer term.

What is required for outcome measurement?

Essentially the idea of an outcome implies measurement at more than one point in time, since an impact or effect upon someone must involve either a change in state, or the prevention of a deleterious change which would have happened without services. This means that outcome measurement is not the same as assessment, although conceivably the difference between two assessments at different times might give a measurement of outcome. Measures to be used must be sensitive to the levels of change expected, otherwise changes will not be detected. This may seem an obvious point but, as will be discussed, well-established measures which are very useful for screening or profiling a population may not be suitable for measuring small changes over time (Fitzpatrick *et al.* 1992a,b). A measurement at one point in time only would have to include a retrospective assessment of change or impact, and would consequently have less credibility as evidence. User satisfaction with services provides a partial exception to this, since it may be viewed as an outcome of services, and logically can only be measured after services are received. However, as the discussion in this review will make clear, the use of satisfaction measures is by no means straightforward or unproblematic, nor is it sufficient for assessing outcomes. Satisfaction is strongly affected by initial expectations, and by the information and beliefs which individuals have about what is possible. In addition, there is potentially a danger that a concentration on satisfaction alone may lead to a failure to take account of the relative importance to the user of different impacts of services.

A number of steps are necessary before it is possible to measure in practice the degree to which service objectives have been achieved. Decisions taken at each step are rarely straightforward and frequently open to argument. What has to be decided is: what is to be measured, how is it to be measured, and how we can attribute observed changes to the actions of service providers? These three questions are considered below.

What is to be measured?

The dimensions or areas of outcome to be measured should be related to the objectives for services (Knapp 1984), and views about the appropriate selection of dimensions are therefore influenced by the values of those with a stake in services. In the case of community care, stakeholders include central and local government, voluntary organizations, service managers, front-line vocational and professional staff, users, carers and the general public. Clearly, there is scope for disagreement about the intended aims of service delivery, although in practice objectives may be vague or unstated, or expressed in general terms which permit a wide variety of interpretations. However, the process of translating objectives into measurable outcomes renders potential conflicts more visible. The following chapters will explicitly consider some of the views of these differing groups, the evidence about conflicts of views, and the question of whether consensus about measurement is a sensible aim. The policy aim of giving people a say implies that the views of users and carers should achieve a new prominence. There is no reason to expect this to be a painless process since the objectives valued by users, professionals and the public may not coincide. As Williams (1986: 5) observes:

> Bluntly stated, most of us working in human services are involved to some extent in keeping people off the streets so that they are not a nuisance to the general public . . . it is likely, therefore, that a serious attempt to represent a consumer's view of services, as opposed to society's, will lead to rather different ideas from those traditionally held on what constitutes quality.

We have come across very few examples of systematic attempts to obtain and compare the views of a range of stakeholders in community care. In considering differing views, the question arises as to whether a genuine consensus can be negotiated, or whether it is best to take a pluralistic approach which recognizes differing objectives and evaluate a given service separately for different interest groups. Alternatively, perhaps the views of different interest groups should prevail in relation to different aspects of the service? Questions about the status of professional knowledge or expertise and user access to information are relevant here. Writing about health care, Donabedian (1992) draws a distinction between the technical task to be performed, the interpersonal exchange, and the 'amenities of care', by which he means the circumstances surrounding the performance of the task and the interpersonal exchange. All of these combined constitute the service. In the context of health care, Donabedian (1992: 247) argues that consumers are the right people to define what is desirable and undesirable in relation to the second and third of these:

> It is their expectations that should set the standard for what is accessible, convenient, comfortable or timely. It is they who should tell us

to what extent they have been listened to, informed, allowed to decide and treated with respect.

Donabedian goes on to argue that, even though professionals may have superior technical knowledge about health interventions, consumers are still able to state their preferences among different possible outcomes, degrees of risk and prospects of amelioration, if they are given sufficient information.

Do these arguments about the primacy of user views apply with equal force to community care? The superiority of professional knowledge about the technical task is probably even less likely to be conceded in social care than in health care, but equally, as we have mentioned, there are public expectations that the behaviour of some groups of service users will be controlled. Even where the primacy of user views would be generally accepted in principle, there can be genuine difficulties posed by problems in communicating with some groups of users, especially those with severe impairment of cognitive functioning: if these cannot be solved then we may have to be content with the measurement of aspects of the person's care and environment, either by observation or through data collected from third parties. However, there is an increasing recognition that people who could give valid opinions have been too easily excluded on these grounds in the past (Simons 1994).

How are the selected dimensions to be measured?

The subsequent question of how to measure the dimensions once they have been selected embodies both technical and value issues. For example, agreement on the importance of a broad area such as empowerment, may turn out to be illusory when consideration is given to what specific observations should be made to measure this. Staff may feel that the freedom to choose furniture and fittings constitutes empowerment whereas users may have in mind the right to choose staff. Within the area of health outcomes, a distinction is often drawn between measures in which items are derived from professional views, and those which are based on users' or patients' views (Fitzpatrick et al. 1992a). Certainly there is evidence of differences of view about what constitutes quality of life between doctors and patients (Slevin et al. 1988), carers and doctors (Blyth 1990) and carers and users (Higginson et al. 1990; Grant 1992). Recognition of this last difference is particularly important if carers are to be used as proxy informants on behalf of service users (Cartwright and Seale 1990). Of course, there may also be differences between professional groups. One example of a concept which may be variously interpreted is independence: this may be measured in terms of physical functioning and mobility, or in terms of autonomy, choice and control – the former set of measurements being seen as reflecting a medical model, the latter as reflecting a social model which is more acceptable to the disability movement.

Many of the following chapters illustrate the range of possible ways in which various domains of outcome have been measured, usually in research. Information on technical issues such as the reliability, validity and sensitivity to change of quantitative measures are also to be found in the literature. However, it will become evident that widely accepted measures do not exist for all domains which stakeholders define as important, and that not all approaches to finding information on outcomes involve quantitative methods.

How are inputs to be specified?

Following Lakhani (1992), it is also necessary to specify exactly the intervention or service being provided, otherwise even if we demonstrate positive outcomes, we will not know what has led to these outcomes. Terms such as 'care management' or 'counselling' have a notoriously wide range of meanings within services and, since different studies reflect different definitions, there have often been a number of inconclusive or apparently contradictory findings about the effectiveness of particular forms of intervention (Smith 1987; Cheetham *et al.* 1992). Given that social care is expected to embrace a wider range of outcomes than health care, potentially including areas such as housing and employment, there are likely to be considerable problems in disentangling the effects of the wide range of inputs which might be expected to achieve such effects. In addition, not all outcomes need be a consequence of intervention at individual level. Legislation to counter discrimination, or to improve access to buildings, may have an impact upon disabled people by removing barriers to achieving a normal life.

Proof of attribution

Even if we are clear about the service inputs and have measured outcomes adequately, there remains the problem of demonstrating that any observed changes are indeed a consequence of the service provided and have not happened for some other reason. Perhaps quality of life is generally improving for people in the specified group, or the changes are only what would be expected over time without any intervention? For research-based evaluations, this concern with attribution leads to the need to find comparison groups, who do not receive the service in question but are otherwise similar. Groups can be randomly allocated to receive or not receive interventions, or statistical methods can be used to make sure that the groups being compared are as similar as possible. Such techniques are useful for one-off research and for evaluating innovations, but are unlikely to be available for monitoring routine practice. As Parker *et al.* (1991) observe, outcome measurement is both dynamic and relative: that is, it is concerned with detecting changes over time and with comparing these changes with some expectation or standard.

Where might standards of comparison come from? They might derive from an ideal of what services might achieve; or perhaps a minimum standard, preferably based on research-based knowledge about what it is possible to achieve in a given situation; or, finally, through comparison with another relevant group. For example, some form of cross-institutional design might be applied (Sinclair and Clarke 1981), whereby information is collected across an authority and comparisons are made between subgroups within the authority, say different teams or geographical areas. In interpreting such data, some effort has to be made to take account of known differences in the likely characteristics of clients or levels of need within these subgroups, before any questions are raised about possible differences in practice influencing outcomes. Standards or methods of comparison assume considerable importance outside a research context.

Another way to tackle the attribution problem at the level of the individual service user may be to ask people directly. It is possible in a practice context to collect information on service inputs, outcomes for the user and their carer (where applicable), and to make some check as to whether those involved have some other explanation for any observed changes, or can specify how the improved outcomes have resulted from services. This suggests a role for a more qualitative investigation. In a study which compared information derived from a structured instrument (the SF36) with that obtained in qualitative interviews, Hill *et al.* (1994) argued that the effects of certain interventions, in relation to continence promotion and mental health, were not detectable with the structured health status measure although, in interview, service users and carers were enthusiastic about the differences that services had made. These effects as reported by service users were masked by overall deterioration due to other conditions, or by increased awareness of other difficulties following an improvement in a state of depression. In another paper, Hill and Harries (1993) identified some of the technical and methodological problems in using the SF36 as an outcome assessment instrument with older people using health services. While Hill and Harris acknowledged that there is a role for structured outcome measures, they concluded that it might be more appropriate to begin by listening to what patients have to say without the constraint of structured questionnaires which have been developed by 'experts', for 'experts'. Together, these reports suggest a considerable role for qualitative research in determining the relevant dimensions of outcome from the user's point of view, identifying unanticipated outcomes, and in providing evidence for attribution in situations where there is no control group for comparison. In addition, in-depth methods may be useful in exploring the

particular reasons underlying any observed differences in quantitative measures of activity or performance across different teams or geographical
areas. Box 1.2 offers a model for examining outcomes in routine practice
and highlights some of the issues that need to be addressed.

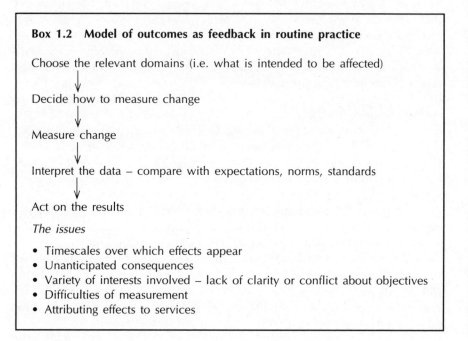

Box 1.2   Model of outcomes as feedback in routine practice

Choose the relevant domains (i.e. what is intended to be affected)

Decide how to measure change

Measure change

Interpret the data – compare with expectations, norms, standards

Act on the results

The issues

- Timescales over which effects appear
- Unanticipated consequences
- Variety of interests involved – lack of clarity or conflict about objectives
- Difficulties of measurement
- Attributing effects to services

Outcome and process

Although we later outline many of the reasons for a shift towards a greater
focus on outcomes for individuals, we do not intend to suggest that consideration of process should consequently be neglected. As will be discussed in later chapters, aspects of process are clearly linked to users' and
carers' expressed dissatisfaction with services. The way in which a service
is delivered, including, for example, staff attitudes, is an integral part of
social care for many service users. As will be outlined in the remainder of
this chapter, some of the avowed objectives of community care policies
for individuals – such as 'having a say in services' or 'improving choice' –
might be interpreted as referring as much to process as to outcomes. While
these may or may not be regarded as ends in themselves, it is clear that any
attempt to evaluate community care would have to consider what would
be evidence of success or failure in achieving these objectives among others.

Having clarified the most widely accepted conceptualizations of outcomes,
we will now consider outcome measurement in relation to community care
policy and practice.

Policy and practice

Community care – social and health care definitions

Our focus in this book is on those policies and services which aim to provide help and support to disabled people to assist them to achieve a normal life in their own home or in a 'homely setting'. It is widely recognized that the majority of such care is provided by family members and, less commonly, by neighbours and friends. These carers as well as users will be important actors in the community care arena. The formal services available take many forms, and the users of services include older people, younger disabled people with physical or sensory impairments, people with learning disability and people with mental health problems. Later chapters will consider each of these groups separately and in more depth. Measures appropriate for residential care environments have not been included, although some of the outcome measures for individuals could be used in residential care, and some measures of quality of life will include details of the physical and social environment. Reviews are available elsewhere of measures specifically suitable for residential care environments, for example, Raynes (1988).

Community care is delivered by a wide variety of agencies including health and social services as well as the voluntary and private sectors. The dividing line between health and social care is not always clear-cut, although some types of assistance are clearly one or the other. The intended outcomes undoubtedly overlap, particularly in relation to such concepts as quality of life. Moreover, health and social services agencies are increasingly examining opportunities to address issues of mutual concern, where the actions of one agency have implications for the other, or where closer collaboration will result in a more effective and more 'seamless' service for users. While joint commissioning offers the potential to address the grey area of overlap between agencies, the improved coordination of separate services can help to ensure that the full range of users' needs will be appropriately addressed. Where agencies are jointly planning services, it makes sense to adopt a joint approach to outcome measurement as well. The issues discussed in this book will be applicable in that area of overlap, but the main focus will nonetheless be on social care. The literature on outcomes in primary health care has been reviewed elsewhere (Wilkin *et al.* 1992); there is also a substantial literature on health-related quality of life (McDowell and Newell 1987; Bowling 1991, 1995). Work on health-related outcomes is substantial in comparison with work on outcomes related to social care, and it will be clear there is much of value to be learned from the health-related literature. However, it is of relevance that those areas in which the most severe practical difficulties have been identified in relation to measuring health outcomes are those where it might be argued the overlap with social care is greatest. Thus, the briefing issued by the UK Clearing House on Health Outcomes (1993: 10) commented:

> There are serious practical difficulties evaluating some types of services. These include problems of measuring outcomes when the service has low level effects, when the start and end of treatment is unclear (outcomes for long courses of rehabilitation or continuous symptom amelioration in chronic conditions), and when several treatments are being conducted simultaneously.

A reading of the voluminous literature on health outcomes and health-related quality of life makes it clear that, despite considerable effort and considerable achievement, there is a very long way to go in developing systems of outcome measurement which will overcome the identified difficulties of ensuring a uniform specification of service inputs, measuring changes in health states, making correct attributions, encouraging systematic outcome measurement in routine practice, and providing and interpreting aggregate information about service users and the general population on a routine basis (Lakhani 1992).

Despite this need for further progress, there is a knowledge base, largely professionally generated, about expected outcomes of at least some aspects of health care. In addition, there are probably ever-continuing, ongoing debates about the relative contributions which can or ought to be made to the evaluation of health care services, and the distribution of health care resources, by patients, the general public, practitioners and managers. There is a research base of studies which enables us to understand lay conceptions of health: what people expect from the health care system, how they do in fact make judgements about health services and how they evaluate medical procedures. We understand much less about what people expect from community care, or what conceptions they might have of the kind of 'normal life' such services should be able to achieve, or what criteria they do, or would, use to evaluate services. What does seem likely is that the boundary between outcome and process will be somewhat less clear-cut, and that people will be less willing to accept the superiority of professional judgements in social care than in health care. The objectives for individuals espoused in the 1989 White Paper *Caring for People* are widely endorsed, although this may reflect the level of generality at which they are expressed. They form a sensible starting point for our discussion of outcome measurement in the context of community care.

Central policy objectives

To what extent can the objectives articulated at policy level be translated into desired consequences for users and carers, and, if they can, are there

accepted ways of measuring these? In conceptual terms, some policy objectives may be achieved without discernible effects on users. For example,
improved value for money might be achieved by producing an unchanged
outcome for users at a lower cost. Other objectives, such as stimulation of
the private sector and a move away from provision by public bodies, may
be seen as ends in themselves but are more usually justified as a means
towards a desirable end for clients, such as increased choice. Promoting
choice and independence for individuals is stated to underlie all the Con-
servative Government's proposals for community care.

The White Paper *Caring for People* lists both client and service-level
objectives. The former are perhaps most clearly reflected in the list of
intentions in paragraph 1.8:

- enable people to live as normal a life as possible in their own homes or
  in a homely environment in the community;
- provide the right amount of care and support to help people achieve
  maximum possible independence, and, by acquiring or re-acquiring basic
  living skills, help them to achieve their full potential;
- give people a greater individual say in how they live their lives and the
  services they need to help them do so.

A 'normal life' is a relative concept. That is, it has to be defined in relation
to what is expected within the society in which a person lives, and may
therefore vary across time and across cultures. Parker *et al.* (1991) have
developed outcome measures for children looked after by a local authority with reference, they say, to the expectations of normal parenting. With
regard to adults, the most comprehensive attempts to operationalize the
idea of a normal life have been in relation to people with learning disability, particularly those discharged from long-stay hospital into community-
based settings (Emerson and Hatton 1994). These measures have been
highly influential but have been subject to attack precisely because they
may apparently uncritically reflect aspects of normal life which are themselves considered to be in need of change (Brown and Smith 1992). For
example, gender stereotyping may be reinforced by expectations that young
women should be encouraged to undertake roles or activities appropriate
for women. Conflict may arise between the principles of choice and the
wish to help people to undertake valued social roles. Nevertheless, as will
be illustrated in Chapter 7, the idea of a normal life in the community has
given rise to a number of accepted dimensions of measurement for people
who have moved from long-stay residential services to alternative services
in the community.

In addition to the objectives of central policy, there will be variations in
objectives as set by local and health authorities. Examples of these may be
gleaned from published Community Care Plans although not all such plans

contain statements of objectives. The SSI Special Study of 25 1993–4 Community Care Plans concluded that 'plans remain weak regarding specification of measurable outcomes and monitoring arrangements' (Project Summary, Department of Health 1994). Equally, much monitoring of local progress from the centre, and the outline of what might be included in community care charters, concentrates on organizational process and structure, rather than on final or client-based outcomes.

Outcomes and the current community care context

A focus on monitoring organizational processes, rather than outcomes for people, may be understandable while new arrangements are being put into place. However, there are a number of compelling reasons for working out systematic ways in which to decide the extent to which benefits for users and carers are being achieved:

• The new arrangements resulting from the NHS and Community Care Act 1990 represent a challenging culture shift for Social Services Departments towards more flexible user-centred services which, it is intended, will better fit the needs of individuals (Audit Commission 1992b). Only outcome measures at user and carer level can give a convincing indication of whether there is a good fit between needs and services.
• Policy statements stress the promotion of independence, user choice and giving people a say in services (Secretaries of State 1989). Given that there may be conflicts of view between users and staff about whether these are achieved, and what should be done to achieve them, it must be important to undertake evaluations which involve the direct expression of views by users and carers.
• As local authorities implement the purchaser–provider split, the increased importance of contracts generates an ever greater necessity to be specific about what is required and what will be evidence of satisfactory performance. In a review of over 70 contracts issued by Social Services Departments, Smith and Thomas (1993) demonstrated that these early contracts rarely contained an indication of specific outcome measures, particularly at user level, although there might be an expressed aspiration towards their development. As likely, however, were broad and abstract statements of worthy objectives such as treating all clients 'with respect'.
• The greater role for authorities in regulation and the enforcement of standards through inspection units, emphasizes the necessity for more sophisticated and detailed expectations about outcomes for individuals than may have obtained hitherto. Sinclair *et al.* (1990: 386) argued:

> The central failure of community care is not the inability to reduce the rate at which old people enter residential care, disturbing though

this is, but the failure to specify and achieve the standards of welfare which old people and their carers in the community should expect.

Standards related to service structure or process need to be underpinned by an understanding of the likely relationships between these and ultimate effects on users or carers. Indeed there is an argument that outcome specifications are preferable to service standards because the former will be less likely to inhibit flexibility and variety of approach.

- There are competing models of how best to undertake such essential processes as care management and interagency collaboration. Consideration of outcomes for users and carers under different models is necessary to improve our understanding of the relative effectiveness of these different models.

Purposes of data collection and appropriate methods

On a routine basis within services, there are three levels at which outcome information relating to individuals may be used, and at each level the information may be needed for a different purpose. These are, first, the individual level, so that the achievement of service goals for an individual can be assessed by front-line workers; second, aggregated outcome data about individuals served, so that comparisons may be made between individuals and groups, or between groups; and, finally, total population level (including information about outcomes for people not served). Population-level outcome information is necessary in order to understand the overall consequences of the distribution of services across the population. If, for example, all resources were devoted to a very few individuals then it might be easy to demonstrate considerable impact on the welfare of recipients, but there might then be many people negatively affected by the lack of services. Such considerations have led the Central Health Outcomes Unit to broaden the definition of outcome to include the effect of 'a lack of' a service or health intervention, since a measure of population outcome requires aggregated information about effects on those who do and do not receive services (Lakhani 1992). In health, such population measures have conventionally included measures of morbidity and mortality, although there are now increasing attempts, such as the *Health of the Nation* initiative, to move towards a broader and more positive conception of health as embodied in WHO definitions. In community care, destinational outcomes, concerned with whether a person is resident in an institution or in ordinary housing in the community, have been used as crude outcome indicators.

Different purposes generate different measurement requirements; for example, individual practice requires flexibility and objective-setting related to the individual's unique combination of needs and circumstances, whereas aggregation for management information requires consistent structuring of a fixed set of information across different cases. The debate about the optimum level of structure for the right purpose has not yet been resolved, and is reflected in a parallel debate about the degree of structure necessary for use in assessment: structured assessments have been criticized for not being sufficiently related to individual needs or aspirations (Kemp and Middleton 1993). However, there is evidence that more needs are identified and met using structured assessments (Nocon 1992), but also evidence of considerable staff resistance to the use of new assessment instruments which were considered to be overstructured and inflexible (Social Services Inspectorate/NHSME 1993b).

We identify in Chapter 9 a number of obstacles to routine outcome data collection relating to individuals, including not only the absence of suitable measures, but also the lack of clarity and the scope for disagreement about service objectives, the deficiencies of existing information systems, the costs of collection, the difficulties of interpretation, and the experience of resistance from staff, based on organizational culture or the values of particular professional groups. MacDonald *et al.* (1992) argue that there is often a resistance to the idea that general objectives for social work can be identified and measured, and that, even where evidence exists about the effectiveness of different aspects of social work practice, this evidence has had little impact on the profession. Cheetham *et al.* (1992) identify a stream of argument within the social work literature which stresses the intangible and unquantifiable nature of therapeutic activity.

Outside a research context, there are few examples of measures of outcome for users and carers being used for routine collection and interpretation within social services. When interviewed for this study, officials from SSI (Policy Division and Inspection Resources Group) and the NHS Executive's Community Care Unit were unable to identify immediately any established examples of good practice within Social Services Departments in this respect, although there was felt to be considerable interest in the possibility of developing suitable measures and methods. For example, health and social services authorities in the North Western Region have produced a set of documents about 'the transition to outcomes-led services' for people with learning disability, in which they argue (North Western Regional Health Authority 1991: 30):

> There are very many existing measures for inputs and for processes . . . But so far, there have been very few measures for outcomes, desirable as they are.

Outcomes and service process

In theory, at least, if the relationship between service characteristics and outcomes for clients is known, then we need only be sure that a service has the required characteristics to be confident that the desired outcomes for service users will be achieved. That is to say, if definitions of service quality are to be valid, they should be underpinned by evidence that the required outcomes will indeed be achieved by the service arrangements recommended. In practice, particular definitions of service quality may be adopted because they are considered to derive from preferred value positions, or to represent the latest professional fashion, rather than because of any demonstrated connection between these particular forms of service provision and superior outcomes for users and carers (Parker *et al.* 1991; MacDonald *et al.* 1992). Parker *et al.* argue that, if routine outcome assessments in child care are to use intermediate outcomes (that is, a measure of what is being done rather than the final impact on the child), then their use must be firmly underpinned by research which investigates and supports the assumed connections between intermediate and final outcomes. It has been argued that the community care changes, unlike those embodied in the Children Act, are not firmly linked into such a foundation (Sinclair 1990). Hughes (1990), in considering the development of suitable quality-of-life measures for older people, comments on the absence of an agreed body of theoretical knowledge of human development in old age, and contrasts this with the well-established and broadly agreed definitions and milestones of normal development for children. The assessment and action records devised by Parker *et al.* (1991: 12) are said to 'specify objectives derived from research on child development and child care practice and link them to actions which have been shown to be necessary for their achievement'.

Is there a sufficient knowledge base to develop a similar system for community care? As the following chapters will indicate, with a few exceptions, studies of community care which have systematically investigated outcomes for users and carers have been concerned with the evaluation of service innovations or deinstitutionalization, rather than the continuing evaluation of routine practice, and have often used institutional care rather than the lives of non-disabled people as an implicit standard of comparison. However, it will be suggested that there is a body of knowledge about the outcomes of specific services, and about outcome measurement, which, however partial or limited, would probably assist managers and practitioners, if it were widely disseminated and used. It has been strongly argued that links between the academic community and managers and practitioners in social care need to be strengthened and improved (Independent Review Group 1994). However, the literature on the diffusion of innovations and on the utilization of research results within health care practice suggests that merely improving dissemination may have little effect on the factors which influence the utilization of research knowledge by professionals in health or social care (MacGuire 1990; Domoney 1993). We will return to this issue in the final chapter.

Conclusions

This chapter has demonstrated that there is a reasonably clear agreed conceptual framework for understanding what is meant by the term 'outcome', and within this framework, despite differences in labelling, an agreed differentiation of the final or client-based outcomes which are the focus of this book. There are many steps to be taken to move from this conceptual framework to the achievement of outcome measures for practice in social care. At this stage, a large number of questions remain to be addressed. Can the stated objectives of community care policy for individuals be measured? Both technical and value-related aspects are involved in addressing this question. For example, is there a technical basis for measurement to be found in research? Can the views of various stakeholders be combined and incorporated in agreed measurements? Are there widely differing ideas about desirable outcomes for different groups of service users? Subsequent chapters will begin to consider these questions. It seems unlikely that the different purposes for which outcome measurement is required can be fulfilled by one kind of measure or one method of measurement.

While recognizing the importance of lessons to be derived from work on health outcomes, it is necessary to sound a note of caution about drawing analogies from such work with an uncritical expectation that they will be appropriate to social care. Much social care is a process rather than a well-defined intervention, the objectives to be achieved are different, and, of particular importance when considering routine practice, the organizational context and culture are also different. The next chapter will consider what is known about emerging practice in Social Services Departments, in relation to areas such as quality assessment and the use of performance indicators, where outcome measurement would seem to be of considerable relevance.

Summary

Outcome is conceptualized as the impact or effect of services on users or carers. This conceptualization generates an understanding of the elements that are required for outcome measurement.

- It is necessary to understand which aspects of a person's state or situation are intended to be affected: is it their psychological well-being, their opportunity for social activities, their everyday functioning?
- Once the appropriate domains have been selected, it is necessary to decide how to measure these areas so that the changes it is hoped to achieve will be detectable.

Although technical and professional knowledge may be useful here, neither of these steps is value-free. There is a range of interested parties, or stakeholders, in community care who may well have different opinions about the selection of domains, and, even if there is an agreement at an abstract level, about a domain, such as independence, there may still remain differences about the way in which such a concept should be operationalized for measurement.

In the research literature, a distinction has been drawn between intermediate and final outcomes, although this sometimes refers to the sequencing through time of outcomes for users or carers, and at other times to a distinction between the ultimate outcomes of the system, those which reflect impact on users, and intermediate changes in service inputs or service quality, which reflect impacts on front-line services. A distinction is also drawn between the measurement of objective and subjective aspects of outcome; that is, between observable aspects of the person's situation – such as how many social contacts they have – and the person's own evaluation of, or response to, such aspects. These two elements are not as closely related as might be hoped. Both objective and subjective aspects need to be measured since there is a balance to be struck between ensuring that individuals receive services which they value, and ensuring a distribution of resources which is seen to be fair in terms of the opportunities given to people in similar situations.

Community care embodies aspects of both health and social care. Although there is a very substantial literature on health outcomes, it seems that these are most fully developed in relation to acute care, and that many of the practical and conceptual difficulties of looking at community care outcomes are common to health and social care. These include the difficulties of assessing the impact of long-term continuing care which may have no particular end-point, and the impact of preventative services, where effects may be long term and there may be considerable problems in attributing effects to services. It may be that social care is expected to embrace a wider range of outcomes than health care, including areas such as material welfare or employment.

In order to see whether intended outcomes are being achieved, it is necessary to consider what the objectives of services are, and how these objectives might be translated into specific measurements at individual level. Central policy gives prominence to ideas about a normal life, maximum independence, achieving individual potential, and giving people a say in services.

In the field of community care, a number of features of the current policy and practice context lead to an increased focus on the question of outcomes for users and carers. These include: the intended shift towards the greater centrality of the views of users and carers; the growth of commissioning and contracting; the greater role for local authorities in the regulation and enforcement of standards; and the continuing need to evaluate and compare different models of care, and to assess service effectiveness.

There are three levels at which outcome information may be collected or reported, and at each level the information may be needed for different purposes. These are:

- The *individual level*, so that the achievement of service goals for individuals can be assessed by front-line workers.
- *Aggregated outcome data* about individuals served, so that comparisons may be made between individuals and groups or between groups.
- *Total population level* (including information about outcomes for people not served), so that the overall effects of the distribution of services may be understood.

In interpreting aggregated data, clear and consistent definitions of what is meant by 'service inputs', such as assessment, day care or care management, have to be applied across the board. If not, then variations in outcomes across different groups who have received, or not received, the services in question will not be readily interpretable. In addition, comparison of aggregated outcome data, say across districts or teams, requires an understanding of differences in population characteristics or overall levels of need, since these may also influence variation in outcomes. The assessment of overall population outcomes requires information about impacts on people who do not receive services. Clearly, the impacts which result from any redistribution of services or resources, say towards those in greatest need, have to be understood if the overall impact of services as they are being operated is to be evaluated.

The existing knowledge base in community care as compared with health care is limited and partial. Even the available and potentially useful research-based knowledge is not considered to be effectively disseminated to, or used by, managers and practitioners in the field.

CHAPTER 2

EMERGENT ISSUES AND PRACTICE IN SOCIAL SERVICES DEPARTMENTS

Introduction

The measurement of outcomes often features either implicitly or explicitly in various activities within Social Services Departments (SSDs). At a broad level, these include quality initiatives, performance measurement and satisfaction surveys. Such work is sometimes linked to tasks resulting from the new community care arrangements such as inspections, service contracting, community care planning, complaints procedures and care management. This chapter will consider the nature of such activities and the opportunities they provide to examine outcomes.

Broad organizational tasks

Box 2.1   Organizational initiatives to measure or improve performance

- Quality assurance
- Performance measurement
- Satisfaction surveys

Practice varies, but:

- The focus is often on activity and process, rather than outcomes
- Users' and carers' involvement is often minimal

Quality

Reasons for the current focus on quality

According to James *et al.* (1992), the current concern with quality derives from four main factors:

- a wish to obtain – and demonstrate – value for money;
- the need to show that policy objectives are being achieved;
- a desire to improve the services available to users; and
- as a means of assisting departmental change.

Such factors reflect broader pressures on public services to account for the way they use public funds and to pay greater attention than previously to service effectiveness and cost-effectiveness. At the same time, users have become more vocal in expressing their own demands, and responsiveness to those demands has become a cornerstone of community care policy.

The responsibility for ensuring better quality services lies with SSD managers. Drawing on Osborne and Gaebler's (1992) reasons for measuring performance, James (1993) notes the advantages of a focus on quality in SSDs:

- what gets measured gets done;
- if you don't measure results you can't tell achievement from failure;
- if you can't recognize failure you can't address it.

Importantly, these statements refer to the impact of service, and not just to the process by which they are delivered. In addition, a focus on quality offers an opportunity to set standards, establish values, manage power and control, and implement change and innovation (James 1992). At the same time, a top–down approach can lead to suspicion that quality is a management weapon, and consequently to resistance to quality initiatives (Kearney and Miller 1994). The history of such initiatives itself often lies in quality control or inspection – reactive procedures that emphasize sanctions rather than the provision of incentives or motivation to improve services (James 1992).

What is quality?

One of the reasons why the concept of quality attracts general approval is that it can be defined in a variety of ways, to suit a number of different purposes. Pfeffer and Coote (1991) outline five broad meanings:

- a reflection of prestige or positional advantage;
- the achievement of standards set by experts;
- a managerial wish to achieve excellence – as measured by user satisfaction;

- empowerment of the service user;
- a democratic approach, based on a wish to achieve commonly agreed goals and meet individual needs – this includes 'fitness for purpose' (derived from the expert approach), 'responsiveness' (from the concern with excellence) and 'empowerment' (the consumerist approach).

A different classification was proposed by Maxwell (1984) in relation to health care. He identified six principal dimensions of health care quality:

- access to services;
- relevance to need (for the whole community);
- effectiveness (for individual patients);
- equity (fairness);
- social acceptability;
- efficiency and economy.

Both sets of definitions include elements that may be difficult or impossible to reconcile. Pfeffer and Coote highlight different philosophical approaches and different interest groups. Maxwell examines the different dimensions of a public service, including its objectives and functions within society, the process of service delivery and outcomes for users. Given the wide range of definitions, Pollitt (1987b) asks what the trade-offs will be between the various elements, both in terms of overall objectives and in relation to the allocation of limited (human and material) resources. The answer will usually depend on the balance of power between stakeholders, which, in the case of publicly funded community care services, is generally weighted in favour of central and local government policymakers.

Consumerism

The increasing emphasis on consumerism nonetheless represents an important countervailing force. According to the National Consumer Council (1987: 1), 'service providers must discover what consumers want and need, then measure their achievements against this standard: ... whatever the economy or efficiency of a service, it has no value if consumers don't want it or can't use it'. Such principles have been endorsed at a political level, where concerns about the accountability and power of public bureaucracies have been reflected in an increased emphasis on the needs and wishes of service users themselves. In practice, however, such an emphasis can take different forms, ranging from the 'customer relations' model, designed primarily to please consumers, to the concept of the 'citizen–consumer' who is empowered to participate at all levels of the policymaking process (Pollitt 1988).

In relation to quality itself, James et al. (1992: 5), writing for the Social Services Inspectorate (SSI), state categorically that 'the primary definition of Quality should be that of the service user not the service provider or service commissioner'. This incorporates the view that quality, 'at its simplest', is about meeting individuals' needs (Warr and Kelly 1992). From a health care perspective, Donabedian (1992) specifically stresses users' unique ability to define what outcomes should be pursued in their own individual cases. In addition, though, he argues for user involvement in all aspects of the definition of quality, from the quality of particular technical tasks, personal interactions, and the circumstances in which tasks are carried out, to the overall shape and quality of services as a whole.

Although the ethos of social services provision endorses the principles of enablement, empowerment and self-determination, its historical and social functions have led to perceptions of service users as social casualties rather than citizen–consumers (Centre for Policy on Ageing 1990). SSD practitioners' belief in their own expertise frequently leads them to devalue the views of users and carers, or to view user self-determination and participation as a threat to their own power (Ellis 1993). Within SSDs as a whole, the introduction of community care planning has been accompanied by injunctions to include users and carers in the planning process. While different user groups themselves have different perceptions of their role, problems have also been experienced in attempting to reconcile the views of users and other stakeholders, such as managerial staff (Wistow and Barnes 1993). James herself noted that the experience of the service user 'can be too easily overlooked' (1992: 6). This has major implications for the measurement of service outcomes.

The focus of quality initiatives

Quality initiatives frequently focus on process, outputs and effectiveness (Berry *et al.* 1985; Davies 1987; Healy and Potter 1987). It is perhaps easier to set standards, establish whether work has been carried out, monitor whether specifications are adhered to, identify defects, quantify products or activities, and measure users' satisfaction, than to determine service effectiveness or outcomes.

Osborne (1992) suggests that the production of welfare approach offers a framework for evaluating both the quality of a service and the quality of life of the service user, as well as for establishing links between them. According to this model, the quality of a service is a function of the relationship between inputs, the service process and outputs. These are mediated by the social environment to produce intermediate outcomes (which Osborne defines as immediate effects on users) and final outcomes (or longer-term impacts). The intermediate and final outcomes represent changes in quality of life.

A first stage of quality control might then focus on the process of service provision and on service outputs. It would examine how those outputs relate to needs ('fitness for purpose') and how users view the process (its 'excellence'). A second stage would be concerned with the relationship between service outputs and outcomes for users. Osborne suggests that needs-based participative planning systems (such as Individual Programme Planning) offer one means of evaluating intermediate outcomes – in relation to the relevance of the outputs to identified needs and progress towards meeting them. Sub-objectives could be measured and aggregated in order to evaluate the effectiveness of the service as a whole. Final outcomes would require evaluation at longer intervals, for instance every two years.

In a discussion about quality, however, Gaster (1991) questions whether the strict separation of process and outcome is always possible. For an agency to respond when users need a service relates to process, yet it also represents an aspect of outcomes for users. The same applies to the stipulation that a service should meet users' wishes. 'Non-technical' aspects of the service process include listening, giving time, empathizing, thinking through and looking for underlying problems, giving information and allowing users to make choices: these aspects, too, reflect the difficulty of establishing where process ends and outcomes begin. Gaster argues that quality initiatives should focus on issues related to service provision, such as accessibility, personal accountability, sensitivity, responsiveness, honesty, the provision of information and a welcoming environment. In contrast to Osborne and Gaebler (1992), with their emphasis on measuring results, Gaster (1995: 117) argues that the difficulties of measuring and interpreting outcomes are such that managers may wish to choose not to attempt this in the first instance. While we would agree that process is an important aspect of quality, we consider that the arguments for a greater focus on final outcomes are compelling.

Quality initiatives within Social Services Departments

One of the central objectives of the new community arrangements, as outlined in the White Paper *Caring for People* (Secretaries of State 1989: para 5.1), was to secure and safeguard the necessary quality of services. There are many examples of quality initiatives within SSDs. In Westminster, evaluation project teams evaluate service quality using a variety of methods: semi-structured interviews, surveys, checklists and observation (James *et al.* 1992). An audit of residential homes has been carried out in Birmingham; in this case, observational techniques were used, in addition to interviews with staff, residents and relatives (James *et al.* 1992). In Lancashire, a quality-of-life instrument was being used to measure user outcomes as part of the local authority's policy for mental health services (Mental Health Social Work Research and Staff Development Unit 1993). In Kensington and Chelsea, a rehabilitation project for people with long-term mental health problems involved users in setting specific objectives, and progress towards these was evaluated at three- to six-monthly reviews; when work with individual users came to an end, they were asked to complete an evaluation form and indicate the ways in which they had or had not been helped.

Quality initiatives can focus on a variety of different issues, depending on who is involved, but they do not necessarily include user input. SSD managers taking part in a workshop, for example, wished to concentrate on assessing the performance of their teams (Kearney and Miller 1994). As part of this process, they identified a need to demystify management information and examine the different languages used by planners and practitioners. The workshop aimed to help them integrate information related to monitoring and evaluation on the one hand, and professional practice on the other.

Other initiatives focus on gathering users' views in order to improve services. Saunders et al. (1992) describe four case studies which involved interviews or questionnaires for users about the services provided and improvements they would like to see. In Humberside, interviews with users provided a basis for developing service standards (Leckie 1994). User and carer forums are becoming increasingly common, both as a means of service evaluation and to achieve specific improvements or service developments (Barnes 1992).

One of the features of quality initiatives is that they examine specific services in detail. They offer an opportunity to identify stakeholders' views of the desired outcomes of individual services, and to establish whether those outcomes are being met. While they may not be suited to routine outcome monitoring, they are appropriate where outcome criteria have yet to be identified or where detailed and focused work is required.

Performance measurement

Given the different meanings of the term 'quality', it is perhaps not surprising that its relationship with performance measurement should be defined in different ways. Wyn Thomas (1990), in a study for the National Consumer Council, presents the two terms sequentially, with performance evaluation providing a basis for improving service quality. On the other hand, both James (1992) and the National Consumer Council (1987) see performance measurement as a way of assessing the quality of a service.

Performance measurement has been defined as (Barnes and Miller 1988: 1):

a coherent collation of information on aspects of services provided and about those needing, seeking or receiving them. The information should constitute a selection of 'measures' which derive from an explicit statement of values and objectives and should relate directly to an assessment of whether these values and objectives are being met.

The National Consumer Council (1987) approach focuses on three principal components: cost, efficiency and effectiveness. In Barnes and Miller's framework, these are expanded into ten broad categories, including needs, objectives, service inputs and their quality, user characteristics, pattern of usage, costs and outcomes (for users, carers and society more generally). Together with a number of sub-categories, these represent a wide-ranging and daunting array of measures. Their review of measures for services for older people is broken down into four categories: policies and objectives, ongoing management information, 'one-off' collection and qualitative measures. It identifies 13 separate policies, based on 30 objectives, with several data sources for each. McLellan's (1992) review of indicators for rehabilitation services offers a similarly extensive range, including data on incidence, prevalence, the environment, broad policies, the quality of interventions, availability of services, problems experienced by individuals, their self-care abilities, quality of life, personal plans and satisfaction with services.

Difficulties arise in determining which aspects of a service to measure, what standards to set, and whose standards to choose (National Consumer Council 1987). The problems arise from the diversity of purposes underpinning performance measurement, and whether it is seen as:

- a means of public accountability;
- a control system, offering early warning of performance which may be falling below expected norms; or
- a developmental aid – part of a learning cycle intended to improve performance.

(Burningham 1990)

Moreover, performance measurement is often seen by service deliverers as an imposition from above, dangerously oversimplified, and providing management with a crude rationale for input minimization (Pollitt 1990). A focus on specific indicators can lead to tunnel vision and 'gaming', with attention being paid to measured activities at the expense of tasks that are less well defined or measured (Burningham 1990; Smith 1992).

Performance measurement in Social Services Departments

SSDs are required to submit management information about their work to the Department of Health and the Chartered Institute of Public Finance and Accountancy (CIPFA). Such information focuses largely on service inputs (such as numbers of staff or expenditure on particular services) or outputs (numbers of residential placements or meals on wheels) (Hoyes et al. 1992). In addition, some authorities have collected information about the community care arrangements introduced in 1993, including the number of comprehensive assessments completed, placements in different types of home and the time that elapses before a placement is made: such indicators are seen as a means of monitoring departmental performance (Warburton 1993). While indicating some destinational outcomes, such information is essentially activity- and process-oriented. Hoyes *et al.* (1992: 41) noted that 'the development of performance measurement of service user outcomes is far from well advanced'.

One feature of most current performance measurement is that it does not involve users: if users are considered at all, it may only be in the indirect form of beneficiaries of any resulting enhanced efficiency (Pollitt 1987a). One reason for this is likely to be the difficulty of quantifying outcomes for users: even assessing the more short-term impact of services (as opposed to 'final' outcomes) calls for a greater clarity of objectives than is generally the case at present (Hoyes *et al.* 1992). A SSD Research and Information Manager has suggested that one possibility might be gradually to introduce quality indicators such as satisfaction measures, attitudinal measures or complaints data into performance data-sets; however, because of the workload involved, it would be necessary simultaneously to reduce the quantity of activity data being collected (Leatherbarrow 1994).

The Citizen's Charter *indicators*

The activity- and input-oriented nature of performance measurement has not been substantially altered by the introduction of the Audit Commission's *Citizen's Charter* indicators for local authority services (1992c, 1993, 1994). The aim of these indicators is to provide information for members of the general public, initially focusing on services within localities, but with comparative information available from 1995. Aware of the costs of information collection, the Commission selected a small number of indicators for each service, generally based on data already being gathered by authorities. For 1994–95, the social services indicators included: demographic information, percentages of people receiving particular services, broad indicators of the frequency of home care provision, broad service recommendations following assessments and an indicator of the time taken to provide equipment costing less than £1000.

The Commission has been complimented for addressing 'an important and hitherto neglected need', namely to provide indicators for the benefit of citizens and which could be used as instruments of public accountability (Harrison 1993). Nevertheless, the indicators have attracted criticism for being imposed on local authorities, not relating to their policy and practice concerns, and being of novelty value only rather than relevant measures of a service (Warburton 1993). Comparative information also creates problems. Variability between areas may result from authorities having different objectives or from their different social and economic environments (Smith 1992). In addition, services may be differently defined in different areas, the fact of service provision does not mean that services are being used efficiently to meet needs, the relative extent of community support networks in a given area can affect the need for public provision and the absence of services can leave informal carers bearing considerable strain. It is certainly possible to defend such indicators on the grounds that they will simply indicate areas which warrant further investigation. However, the array of local factors underlying the level of provision of a particular service is potentially so complex that one SSD Principal Research and Information Officer concluded that, in respect of the *Citizen's Charter* indicators, 'most indicators don't indicate anything!' (Miller 1994). He added that, while indicators might purport to offer advantages such as a basis for planning, improved practice or information for consumers (Gaster 1991), such advantages are more apparent in theory than in reality. The disadvantages and dangers, on the other hand, are numerous: poor data quality, a dominance of the measurable over the important, the cost of data collection, a lack of staff commitment and a lack of user involvement (Gaster 1991). If accurate and useful information is to be provided, it would be necessary to adopt a more detailed and wide-ranging approach (Barnes and Miller 1988).

The Audit Commission, for its part, has stated that it does not wish to examine individual services in 'excessive' detail (1992c: 3); rather, it seeks to focus on issues that would be of general interest to citizens. Although it accordingly commissioned research to identify those aspects of local services that the public considered important, the work of SSDs was excluded because of 'difficulties of confidentiality in interviewing social services clients' (private communication). The social services indicators themselves do not include either an assessment of outcomes for users or any feedback from users about the quality or effectiveness of services.

Local community care charters

The performance indicators are just one element of the *Citizen's Charter* initiative. Another part of the initiative took the form of local community care charters, which SSDs were required to produce in 1995. The aim of these was to lay down standards for the provision of services. Some authorities had already specified service standards, as a means of making known what types and levels of services users and carers could expect. The charters that SSDs were now required to produce, however, were generally broader in their scope: they should, for instance, specify standards for the provision of information, assessment and care planning, the involvement of users and carers, complaints procedures and performance monitoring. Detailed standards were to be worked out locally in consultation with users, carers and other interested parties, and were to reflect local concerns and priorities. Department of Health guidance noted that the broad *Citizen's Charter* principles reflected some of the central concerns of the new community care arrangement, such as focusing on users and carers, ensuring that services respond to their needs, and providing diversity and choice; to that extent, therefore, community care charters were as much a part of those arrangements as of the *Citizen's Charter* initiative.

The guidance suggested that performance standards might include aspects of timeliness, reliability, availability, choice and quality. It added that standards should, wherever possible, be in a form that could be quantified. The main focus in the guidance, however, was on process. In practice, some SSDs did specifically refer to outcomes when preparing local charters. A draft charter prepared by Wiltshire SSD, for example, referred to users and carers being encouraged to comment on the outcome of the service received, and audit being both user- and carer-led and focused on outcomes for service users. The extent to which local charters provided an opportunity to measure outcomes thus depended on their specific content. Where outcomes were mentioned, the need to monitor performance would provide a reason for demonstrating what outcomes were in fact being achieved.

Satisfaction surveys

One way in which SSDs have sought to incorporate a user dimension into performance monitoring has been through the use of satisfaction surveys (Barnes and Miller 1988; Alaszewski and Manthorpe 1993). In addition to being a means of evaluating service quality, satisfaction is seen as an outcome measure in its own right, being related to improvements in users' well-being and thus to service effectiveness (Locker and Dunt 1978; Fitzpatrick 1991; Donabedian 1992). It can also indicate any service changes that may be needed (Locker and Dunt 1978).

The results of satisfaction surveys do, however, need to be treated with caution. Box 2.2 summarizes some of the problems that may arise. Results from such surveys do need to be treated with caution. In both health and social care, high satisfaction levels have often been reported. Poor survey design is sometimes responsible for this: a cursory question about whether a user is satisfied or not is likely to elicit an equally perfunctory response (Donabedian 1992). Public and private accounts may differ; users may be unwilling to criticize 'free' services; they may fear that complaints may lead to the withdrawal of services; their judgements may be influenced by their views about individual staff; long waits for a service may be forgotten once the service has been provided; and some users will give answers designed to please the questioner (Huxley and Mohamad 1991; Allen *et al.* 1992; Barnes 1992; Judge and Solomon 1993; Wilson 1993).

Research suggests that satisfaction levels are highly correlated with expectations (Linder-Pelz 1982): indeed, it would seem reasonable that satisfaction should depend on whether users' wishes have been met. However, the relationship between expectations and satisfaction is problematic (Calnan 1988). In the field of health care, some users have no expectations or may

---

Box 2.2   Problems with satisfaction surveys

Broad issues
- General questions may fail to distinguish between views about specific aspects of services
- Questions may not reflect the issues of importance to users

Responses
- Respondents may be unwilling to criticize 'free' services
- Respondents may fear that complaints will lead to withdrawal of services
- Judgements about services may be influenced by views about individual staff
- Retrospective questions may fail to uncover details of past experiences
- Respondents may give answers designed to please the questioner

Relationship between expectations and satisfaction
- People may not have clear expectations
- Expectations will vary between individuals: basing provision on expectations leads to inequity
- People make distinctions between an acceptable level of service and a subjective sense of what they deserve
- People distinguish between a preferred, ideal service and lower expectation of what may be reasonably expected in reality
- Dissatisfaction may only be expressed if there is a gross discrepancy between expected standards and actual experience
- People's views vary in concreteness and specificity
- Expectations change as a result of receiving a service
- Satisfaction is not correlated with beneficial outcomes

---

be uncertain what to expect. Where they do have expectations, these may be determined in part by prior experiences and the experiences of others, but also by individual definitions of what is an acceptable level of service and a subjective sense of what they deserve (Wilkin *et al.* 1992). A distinction is often made between a preferred, ideal, service and the lower expectation of what may reasonably be expected in reality (Locker and Dunt 1978). Satisfaction may then relate just to the achievement of a minimum standard and, indeed, dissatisfaction may only be expressed if there is a gross discrepancy between that expected standard and actual experience (Wilkin *et al.* 1992). A further difficulty with expectations is that different users' expectations will vary in concreteness and specificity; they may also change as a result of the experience of receiving a service (Locker and Dunt 1978). The retrospective appraisal of expectations can thus be difficult. A prospective approach, on the other hand, runs the risk of influencing expectations – and potential satisfaction – as a result of question content (Huxley and Mohamad 1991).

Another important issue concerns the relationship between satisfaction and outcome. Some satisfaction ratings relate primarily to the quality of contact, not outcome (Hall *et al.* 1988; Huxley and Mohamad 1991). Locker and Dunt (1978) found that 10 per cent of the people they interviewed required more help, but only 2 per cent were dissatisfied with the current level of provision. Davies *et al.* (1990: 113) examined users' overall satisfaction as well as service impact and reported that satisfaction was not correlated with other benefits: some users appeared to derive benefit from services without being satisfied, and vice versa. They concluded that 'consumer satisfaction is not a good guide to whether some of the broader aims of social services provision are being achieved'.

High levels of satisfaction can thus be misleading and can lead to the provision of inappropriate services that may not adequately meet users' or carers' needs (Allen *et al.* 1992). The danger is heightened by the fact that current service users may be atypical of all people with particular needs: others may not have been offered a service in the first place, may have refused it if it was not acceptable or appropriate to them, or may have ceased using it (Davies *et al.* 1990). Not least, care is required in the way surveys are carried out and interpreted. Users may be both satisfied with some parts of a service but dissatisfied with others and it is impossible to reflect this in a single question. Equally, changes in overall satisfaction levels may be due to a cumulative shift in all component aspects or to a large shift in just one aspect (Carr-Hill *et al.* 1989). And satisfaction with specific elements of, say, residential care does not mean that users are satisfied with residential care as a way of life (Cheetham *et al.* 1992).

A further problem with satisfaction surveys is that they are often based on providers' agendas, with little or no opportunity for users to specify what issues are in fact important to them (Wyn Thomas 1990). Yet if users are to be asked to evaluate either the quality of care or the extent to which needs are met, they must be able to define the relevant issues and criteria themselves (Locker and Dunt 1978; Carr-Hill *et al.* 1989; Wilson 1993). It is for this reason that a more qualitative, interactive approach is often recommended (Aharony and Strasser 1993; Judge and Solomon 1993; Williams 1994). Consultation projects, for instance, can offer an opportunity for reflection and discussion, enable difficult subjects to be discussed and provide full and detailed responses to services (Walker 1991; Barnes 1992).

The final issue concerns the precise reason why satisfaction surveys are carried out. It is not uncommon for such surveys to be mere organizational rituals, with few implications for practice and frequently intended to justify the existing pattern of services (Wyn Thomas 1990; Michie and Kidd 1994). While they may enable organizations to state they are both evaluating services and 'involving' users, they are essentially an 'add-on', rather than an integral part of service planning and provision.

Despite the apparent attractiveness of satisfaction surveys, they must be approached with great caution. It is often far from clear what is being measured (Carr-Hill 1992); in particular, expressed satisfaction has to be distinguished from views about service outcomes (Shaw 1984). For the information provided by satisfaction surveys to be of value, it is essential that the issues they address should have been clearly identified and that the questions be shown to produce valid and reliable answers. Even so, focusing on satisfaction alone is not a valid short-cut to the measurement of outcomes.

The new community care arrangements

Some potential opportunities for defining and measuring outcomes within the new community care arrangements are shown in Box 2.3.

Box 2.3   Potential opportunities for defining and measuring outcomes within the new community care arrangements

- Community care plans
- Contracts
- Inspection
- Care management assessments

Community care plans

Quality initiatives, performance measurement and satisfaction surveys pre-date the new community care arrangements that were implemented between 1991 and 1993, though in many cases they were influenced by those changes. The new arrangements did, however, introduce a number of additional organizational tasks which potentially offer some scope for outcomes measurement.

One of those tasks is the production of community care plans. According to *Caring for People*, these plans are expected to set out strategic objectives and priorities sufficiently clearly to enable performance to be monitored and assessed (Secretaries of State 1989: para 5.6). In practice, however, many plans have focused on descriptions of services and statements of principle rather than specifying clear objectives that could be monitored in practice (Hardy *et al.* 1993). Global long-term aims perhaps have to be couched at a high level of generality, for example 'assisting people to achieve the best possible circumstances and quality of life' (Avon 1993–94 Community Care Plan: 6). Where targets are set, these typically relate to specific services, such as 'to set up a family placement scheme':

it is rare for targets to be linked to any intention to measure specified out-comes for service users. Some objectives, such as 'to improve awareness of carers' needs, especially in local and health authorities' (Bradford 1993–94 Community Care Plan: 23), would not in themselves necessarily lead to improved outcomes for users and carers, but there is perhaps an implicit expectation that improved awareness on the part of practitioners may lead to better outcomes for carers.

Some authorities are now seeking to transform their community care plans into commissioning documents that will form a basis for service con-tracting: this may offer an opportunity to both specify and monitor outcomes in more detail. Such a transformation, however, is likely to be a slow and complex process. In the meantime, it is possible to look at the current con-tracting process for evidence of outcome specification and evaluation.

Contracts

The White Paper stated that the introduction of contracting would assist in the monitoring of social care services (Secretaries of State 1989: para 5.15). Subsequent guidance noted that service specifications should include details of both quantity and quality, and how these would be monitored (Department of Health 1990: para 4.19). Information about quality could be obtained from monitoring existing users' satisfaction with services, from the complaints procedures, inspection units and individual assessments (para 4.18).

A study of 70 SSD contracts nonetheless found that practice was very variable (Smith and Thomas 1993). A majority of the contracts focused primarily on service inputs and descriptions of the services to be provided. Others were output-oriented, specifying, for instance, the number of users to be served. Aspirations for quality of service process were typically ex-pressed in very general terms, with a resultant lack of clarity about how contract success could be measured. An example of this was that users 'will have dignity respected in every possible way at all times'. Other con-tracts supported their basic aims with more detailed statements about how those aims might be translated into action: residents of older people's homes, for instance, would be encouraged 'to do as much as possible for them-selves and others, including carrying out simple daily tasks'. While such statements still remain at a fairly broad level, it is questionable whether more specific, measurable objectives can be specified without focusing on the specific needs of individual users.

Ninety per cent of the contracts referred to monitoring. However, this often related to overall contract performance rather than to outcomes for individual users, whether in relation to the contracts themselves or to indi-vidual care plans. While surveys, interviews and user forums were mentioned as means of obtaining user feedback, the documentation was generally unclear about who was responsible for this: inspection units, contracting teams, care managers, or – one might add – research and information units or providers themselves. The authors also noted that monitoring requires considerable time and resources, appropriate systems were still in the process of development, and there was a discrepancy between statements about the monitoring of service quality and the lack of such monitoring in practice. The need to specify quality and outcome indicators represents a major task for purchasers.

Inspection units

Among the first aspects of the NHS and Community Care Act 1990 to be implemented was the establishment of inspection units. One of the principal aims of such units is to evaluate the quality of care provided and the quality of life experienced in residential care homes (Department of Health 1990: para 5.6). Additional optional functions include the development of quality assurance programmes and the inspection of other SSD services, such as domiciliary support (para 5.14).

Residential care

The SSI has produced a number of guidance documents which could be used by inspection units and SSD managers when evaluating standards in residential homes (Social Services Inspectorate 1990a,b) or in home support services (ibid.: 1990c, 1993a). In a section on quality of life in residential homes for older people, the guidance notes the importance of user satisfaction (ibid.: 1990a). It suggests that the relationships between the resources and activities described as 'residential care' and quality of life as measured by user satisfaction are complex, and that obtaining an accurate picture of users' views can be difficult. Nevertheless, it specifies some aspects of care that can be monitored: these include comfort, security, privacy, company and interesting activities.

The guidance on residential care for people with a physical impairment extends the discussion of quality of life to include 'consumer rights, needs and satisfaction' (Social Services Inspectorate 1990b). It emphasizes the need to listen to what users have to say, and an appendix lists a number of issues concerned with aspects of daily living and satisfaction with the care setting: these are intended for use as an interviewing guide during the course of inspection. The guidance also includes a section on assessment and review, and states that reviews should take place periodically to ensure that needs are met as circumstances change (ibid.: para 6.6). The main focus here, though, is on process rather than content: details of individual outcomes would be considered in relation to individual care plans rather than the inspection process. The same applies to the method as a whole: while it is broad ranging and offers a means of structuring discussions, its principal objective is the evaluation of facilities as a whole, not outcomes for individual users.

Nevertheless, some inspection units have been instrumental in developing standards for residential care that include specific indicators for evaluating the quality of care. In Leeds, for example, the inspection pro forma includes questions about choice of meal-times and in the purchase of clothing, as well as links between a home and the local community (Warburton 1993). Trafford SSD (1993), for its part, lists 178 'outcome criteria', grouped around 28 separate standards. Specific criteria include: choice about when to get up, the availability of help in making and receiving telephone calls and satisfaction with the help given to maintain personal hygiene. Such features are important measures of service quality, but they primarily relate to process criteria. The extent to which they may also be considered as outcome criteria for individual users depends largely on the definition of outcome. They are not measures of quality of life, morale, life satisfaction or well-being. On the other hand, they are based on five core values (independence, choice, fulfilment, dignity and privacy) which themselves reflect the objectives of *Caring for People*. The 178 outcome criteria, as outlined above, represent a means of determining whether these values underpin the service provided and whether the objectives are being met.

Home support services

As in the case of residential care, the SSI's earlier document on the inspection of home care services focuses primarily on aspects of the service provided, although it does include a systematic approach to the assessment of users' functional and self-care abilities (Social Services Inspectorate 1990c). A later handbook (ibid.: 1993a) adopts a much broader approach. As in the example above, it specifies the key values that should underpin the provision of home support services, including autonomy and independence of decision-making, choice of lifestyle, respect for the intrinsic dignity of each person and privacy from unnecessary intrusion.

The next step is to ensure that such values are translated into practice, and in a way that can be monitored. The guidance states that SSDs have to be clear about the service specifications and quality standards they will use. Service principles accordingly include user control, being able to choose from different service options, and making decisions about daily routines and lifestyles (Social Services Inspectorate 1993a: 10). More detailed criteria include: whether users can choose what to wear, how to prepare food, whether tasks are performed at times that suit the user, respect for personal choice (for instance about having a bath or shower, hairstyle or make-up), respect for users' wishes to carry out certain tasks themselves and the right of the user to refuse help.

While such issues again relate primarily to the process of service provision, they are designed to reflect the principles set out in *Caring for People*. According to the SSI, the success of services is itself to be judged on the basis of user satisfaction with results (1993a: 27). Data are to be regularly collected about both user satisfaction and users' expressed needs and preferences: this will form an integral part of performance review and indicate both the quality of services and the extent to which they respond to local needs. In addition, individual reviews (following on from initial assessments and forming part of the care management process rather than inspection itself) will provide a basis for monitoring the extent to which previously identified needs and objectives have been met. Establishing that such reviews are taking place represents one element of the inspection process.

Complaints

The new community care arrangements also included the introduction of complaints procedures, whereby users or their representatives can make complaints about the quality or nature of services (Department of Health 1990: para 6.10). Such procedures are seen as an additional means of monitoring performance and the extent to which service objectives are being achieved. While the establishment of formal procedures does make it easier for complaints to be made, they are only a partial indicator of quality and a poor measure of outcomes. Complaints are generally only made when services fall well below a minimally acceptable standard and, even then, not all users will feel sufficiently emboldened to make a complaint. Their high threshold and unsystematic nature preclude their use for evaluation. They are, in addition, more likely to be concerned with aspects of process rather than with effectiveness or outcomes. Not least, they principally reflect dissatisfaction with a service.

Care management and assessment

The new care management and assessment system, on the other hand, is specifically concerned with identifying and meeting individuals' needs for community care services. To be truly effective, this approach must include the regular review of needs to establish whether initial objectives are being or have been met, to identify any changes in needs, and to monitor the quality of services provided, including users' and carers' views (Department of Health 1990: para 3.52). Given that the initial assessment will have set a baseline, the reviews offer the potential to measure community care outcomes.

The extent to which this potential can be realized depends on the way the initial assessment is carried out and the amount of information recorded. Assessment procedures differ widely, though most have some hierarchy of complexity. Some, for example, use a three-tier assessment process which includes a basic screening process, a 'core' assessment, and a more detailed, comprehensive procedure (Social Services Inspectorate/NHSME 1993b). Hoyes *et al.* (1992) describe one SSD's intention to use its detailed assessment form to generate outcome scores for individual users. The form included 11 assessment areas (such as domestic activities and mobility), each of which was broken down into more specific elements and graded into five categories reflecting the extent of problems faced by individual users. Even where no improvements were likely in one area, such as health status, objectives could nonetheless be set in others. Periodic reassessment would enable comparisons to be made and outcomes measured.

A report by the SSI and NHS Management Executive (1993b) noted a general trend away from detailed assessment formats. Many authorities had initially devised complex and comprehensive assessment documentation which was time-consuming to complete (if it was completed at all) and often included large sections that were irrelevant to individual users. The report endorsed the move towards either more specialist documentation or simpler approaches which allowed users to specify their needs. At the same time, the report noted that assessors often adopted a service- rather than a needs-led approach to assessment, so that users' needs were not clearly recorded.

The way in which needs are recorded has major implications for any subsequent review and determination of whether those needs have been met. A general statement of objectives in terms such as 'supporting a person at home', for instance, does not provide a sufficiently clear baseline for the measurement of outcomes. Such measurement would ideally require the use of a validated and reliable instrument at both the initial assessment and subsequent review, in order to indicate any changes in say, a user's or carer's well-being, quality of life or ability to maintain an independent life-style. Instruments of this sort do not, however, currently form part of assessment procedures and the move away from structured approaches makes their adoption increasingly less probable. It could be argued that a general statement about whether a person's needs in a particular area have been met, would be a sufficient means of monitoring a service's effectiveness. However, such an approach remains subjective: it is unclear how the initial assessment was made, what precise objectives the service is meant to achieve, or the basis on which a judgement is made that needs have or have not been met. Nor does it indicate what specific types of services need to be planned and provided to meet specific types of needs.

A further practical problem concerns the extent to which reviews are carried out at all. The Social Services Inspectorate/NHSME report noted there were difficulties in undertaking these, largely because of the time required and the work pressures arising from the new community care arrangements. As a result, reviews were sometimes carried out by telephone or by questionnaire – although the report did not specify the form of such questionnaires. Other information from individual SSDs indicates that some have used satisfaction surveys to focus on the effectiveness of the assessment process, rather than formally collating data about outcomes from reviews themselves. The reason for their choice is a suspicion that care managers might be likely to bias the results if they were to carry out evaluations of their own work. Such a consideration would certainly be valid where the evaluation uses an open-ended format, is concerned with the quality of the assessment process itself, allows the evaluator to judge the effectiveness of the service provided, and – above all – does not involve the use of instruments with a proven record of reliability. However, the questionnaires that have been used have provided only a limited amount of information about outcomes. In one case, the relevant question asks, 'Do you now get the help from Social Services that you need?', with space for further comments. The draft interview schedule produced by another SSD asks, 'Has your life changed as a result of the new services?' and 'If yes, how?'. It has to be acknowledged, though, that the primary purpose of such surveys is to obtain users' views about the quality of the services provided, rather than to assess outcomes as such.

A different approach was adopted by the Social Work Research Centre at the University of Stirling in a study of the outcomes of different models of care management in four regions in Scotland (Social Work Research Centre 1993). The monitoring instrument that was used was a case recording form that summarized the identified areas of need (for both users and carers) and the issues to be addressed in the care plan. The form was completed by the care manager, and a second form, completed nine months later (or at closure, if earlier), would establish what changes had occurred. Interviews were also being carried out at that stage with users and carers, and individual packages of care were costed. The forms themselves were being completed by care managers in addition to their own documentation.

It remains to be seen whether authorities will wish to use such an approach to monitor the effectiveness of their services once the research project comes to an end. Not only does the collection of data call for additional work on the part of care managers: its collation also requires technology that can handle such data, and research or information staff with sufficient time to input and analyse it. Evidence from a Social Services Research Group (1994) workshop has suggested that much of the time of SSD research and information staff was spent gathering information on the Audit Commission's performance indicators: existing resources would reportedly be insufficient to undertake the routine collation of assessment or review data.

Conclusions

This chapter has examined a number of quality and performance initiatives in SSDs, as well as the systems and procedures introduced by the new community care arrangements. Outcome measurement is potentially a central component of many of these procedures and, as the Audit Commission (1992a) has pointed out, such measurement is ultimately the only way of assessing the impact of the community care changes. Yet, although there are many opportunities for developing outcome measurement, in practice SSDs have made slow progress in developing such work. It is all too easy to adopt approaches such as measures of activity or satisfaction surveys, despite the problems inherent in interpreting these or relating them to service impact or the quality of users' and carers' lives. Even before the technical aspects of developing more appropriate measures can be considered, however, conceptual clarity is required about the nature of outcomes, and this is in itself a major task.

These first two chapters have considered the objectives of central government and SSDs in implementing the new community care arrangements. However, one of the main objectives of the new system is to provide a service that is responsive to the needs of individual users and carers: this should, therefore, provide a basis for outcome measurement, too. Chapter 3 will consider the views of users and carers about community care and how their needs might best be met.

Summary

Social Services Departments have carried out a good deal of work on quality and performance measurement, both of which might offer some potential to examine community care outcomes. The focus of much of the work, however, has been on activities and processes, not outcomes: this is the case, for example, with the *Citizen's Charter* indicators. It is also largely true of satisfaction surveys. These do sometimes seek to obtain users' and carers' views of the outcomes of, say, assessments; nevertheless, the precise meaning of satisfaction is often unclear, and satisfaction surveys offer a poor substitute for a more systematic evaluation of the extent to which social care needs have been met.

The new community care arrangements have introduced a further range of tasks which could play a part in the measurement of outcomes. Community care plans could state objectives in a way that could be closely monitored and evaluated. Service contracts could specify the outcomes to be achieved. Inspection units could monitor those outcomes. And the care management and assessment process could both identify needs in the first instance and subsequently review whether those needs have been met.

Our literature review and discussions have failed, however, to uncover any evidence that these processes are in fact being used to evaluate outcomes. While the assessment and review process may initially appear to offer an opportunity to develop further work on outcomes, the variability in assessment formats and practice means that valid and reliable outcome data may be hard to obtain.

Further reading

Barnes, M. and Miller, N. (eds) (1988) Performance measurement in personal social services. *Research, Policy and Planning*, 6(2): 1–47.
   Sets out a model of performance measurement which incorporates users' views, service information and quality issues. Suggests a range of qualitative and quantitative indicators that might be used.
Connor, A. and Black, S. (eds) (1994) *Performance Review and Quality in Social Care*. London: Jessica Kingsley.
   A range of essays, including discussions of performance review, inspections and complaints procedures. Gives examples of quality assurance and of user and carer involvement in service planning and evaluation.
Ellis, K. (1993) *Squaring the Circle: user and care participation in needs assessment*. York: Joseph Rowntree Foundation.
   Examines the extent to which disabled people and carers are involved in needs assessment. Gives examples of practitioners failing to allow users and carers to define their needs.
James, A., with Brooks, T. and Towell, D. (1992) *Committed to Quality: quality assurance in Social Services Departments*. London: HMSO.
   Discusses the background to quality assurance in personal social services and reviews recent initiatives. Offers suggestions for developing quality assurance systems.
Social Services Inspectorate (1993) *Developing Quality Standards for Home Support Services*. London: HMSO.
   Sets out key principles for the provision of home support services and suggests quality standards to be used in service evaluation.
Williams, B. (1994) Patient satisfaction: a valid concept? *Social Science and Medicine*, 38(4): 509–516.
   Reviews the development of satisfaction surveys. Argues that such surveys generally fail meaningfully to ascertain service users' experiences and perceptions.

CHAPTER 3

SERVICE USERS' AND CARERS' VIEWS ABOUT COMMUNITY CARE

Introduction

The new community care arrangements recognize that the earlier system for the provision of social care was flawed in a number of ways: services failed to be matched to individuals' needs, users lacked choice, services encouraged dependence and service provision was inadequate for many people. Where users and carers have had the opportunity to share experiences and reflect on the system's shortcomings, they have often produced wide-ranging critiques of services, as well as charters of rights and blueprints for community care provision. Their views of desirable outcomes provide a set of criteria against which services can be evaluated.

The importance of users' and carers' views is highlighted in *Caring for People*. At an individual level, people should have 'a greater individual say in how they live their lives and the services they need to help them do so' (para 1.8). Social Services Departments (SSDs) are also expected to involve service users and carers in the planning process (Department of Health 1990). The Social Services Inspectorate (SSI) has suggested, indeed, that the rationale for the reorganization of services is 'the empowerment of users and carers' (Social Services Inspectorate/SWSG 1991: 9). This is a much more radical change of direction than earlier references to consultation and participation. As the SSI points out:

> Instead of users and carers being subordinate to the wishes of service-providers, the roles will be progressively adjusted. In this way, users and carers will be enabled to exercise the same power as consumers of other services. This redressing of the balance of power is the best guarantee of a continuing improvement in the quality of service.

It has to be recognized that the interests or wishes of users and carers may not always coincide. A range of research studies have suggested potential and actual areas of conflict within families, around issues such as the ability of a disabled person, or a carer, to live an independent life (Lewis and Meredith 1989; Qureshi and Walker 1989; Grant 1992). For care managers, the negotiation of differing views held by different family members may be a key skill. In some cases, though, professionals may see themselves as working to supersede carers (Twigg and Atkin 1994). On the other hand, it is important not to assume that users and carers will hold conflicting views in all cases. Wertheimer (1991) reported that users and carers at a joint conference were largely in agreement with one another. Roberts *et al.* (1994) found that older service users rated the meeting of carers' needs more highly as an objective than did professional health service staff.

This chapter will examine both the nature of user empowerment and the views of users and carers about community care in general and specific services in particular.

The nature of empowerment

Box 3.1   Dimensions of empowerment

- A market or democratic approach: exit or voice
- Empowerment as a process or a goal
- Individual or collective

Hirschman (1970) distinguished between two main forms of empowerment: exit and voice. 'Exit' refers to the power that consumers can exert over providers through the possibility of transferring their business to alternative providers if they are dissatisfied with the service they receive. This is broadly compatible with a 'market' approach; it depends, however, on the availability of alternative sources of provision. 'Voice', on the other hand, refers to the ability of consumers to exert influence over a service provider – for instance, if they wish a service to be changed or modified in some way. This 'democratic' approach is also a means whereby users might seek to influence the overall pattern of public services (Taylor *et al.* 1992).

A further important distinction is between empowerment as a process and as a goal in its own right. As an aspect of process, it relates to interaction between users and professionals, with users being given choices, opportunities for redress, a voice in the design of individual care plans, and support, for instance in the form of information and advocacy (Taylor *et al.* 1992). It also includes having a voice in broader service planning. As a goal in its own right, empowerment refers to people's more general ability to take control of decisions affecting their lives, especially where their past experiences have been of professionals making decisions for them. Again, this applies at both an individual and an agency level. Such empowerment will often be a long-term process.

The new community care arrangements encompass aspects of both exit and voice, with empowerment as both process and a final goal. *Caring for People* sets out the objective of people having 'a greater say' in services; it emphasizes the need for users to have choice, advocates the promotion of independence, and calls for a community care system which is needs-rather than service-led and which respects users' expressed needs and wishes. All these objectives are fundamental aspects of empowerment (Stevenson and Parsloe 1993).

One approach to measuring user empowerment in community care is illustrated by the 'ladder of empowerment' (Hoyes *et al.* 1993), based on Arnstein's (1969) ladder of participation. The 'top' of the ladder reflects the 'highest' level of empowerment (see Box 3.2). The ladder provides a means of establishing the extent to which users are genuinely empowered under the new community care arrangements. Current evidence indicates that the level of empowerment is still low, both for individual users and in users' collective involvement in service planning (Bewley and Glendinning 1994; Lamb and Layzell 1994). The specific issues arising in respect of individual and collective empowerment will now be considered in more detail.

Box 3.2   'Ladder of empowerment'

HIGH   Users have the authority to take decisions
         Users have the authority to take selected decisions
         Users' views are sought before decisions are finalized
         Users may take the initiative to influence decisions
         Decisions are publicized and explained before implementation
LOW   Information is given about decisions made.

Individual empowerment in assessment and care management

The assessment of need forms the basis of community care services for individual users. *Caring for People* does not, however, indicate how professionals' and users' potentially different definitions of need should be reconciled. While assessments should 'take account of the wishes of the individual and his or her carer' (para 3.2.6), it is the professional care managers who are responsible for both assessment and the design of care packages. There has certainly been a tendency for professional staff to place more emphasis on their own expertise than on users' views (Ellis 1993; Hoyes *et al.* 1994). Assessments have also been criticized for being humiliating and for focusing on incapacity rather than on disabled people's abilities (Lamb and Layzell 1994). Others have commented that assessments primarily involve the completion of forms and gathering of information, which similarly enforce a feeling of dependency (Cale 1993). Communication problems can be caused by a failure to address language or environmental barriers.

The choices available to users are often limited. This partly arises from existing patterns of service provision and the finite nature of the resources available (Taylor *et al.* 1992). A focus on block contracts further reduces the possibility of individually-designed packages (Common and Flynn 1992; Hoyes *et al.* 1994). Care managers, for their part, may be unaware of the options that exist, or of ways of meeting users' needs (Keep and Clarkson 1994; Morris 1994). Pressure to ration scarce resources can act as a barrier to recording or responding positively to users' expressed needs (Ellis 1993; Stevenson and Parsloe 1993). On the other hand, some care managers are concerned that the new system focuses too much on quantifiable services, and that a bureaucratic, mechanistic approach is failing to address people's needs fully, for instance in relation to emotional support or counselling (Hoyes *et al.* 1994). All too often, users receive 'off-the-shelf' services; yet, even then, simple needs are still not always met (Baldock and Ungerson 1994). Many users remain sceptical of their ability to influence the services they can receive. One respondent in Lamb and Layzell's (1994: 33) study suggested that 'it is not what you as a person wants [*sic*], it is what they say you will have'.

Some social services authorities are now encouraging users to state their needs themselves or to carry out self-assessments (Social Services Inspectorate/NHSME 1993a,b). Unsupported self-assessment, however, can too often lead to an understatement of needs (Kestenbaum 1993). If users are to exercise real control in their lives and have a voice in the way their needs are identified and met, it is incumbent upon care managers to listen to people and not just complete checklists (Hughes 1993; Smale *et al.* 1994). The amount of information given to users, the choices of services available and the degree of control users can exercise over the decisions that are made, all contribute to their empowerment in determining how their needs are to be met (Morris and Lindow 1993; Stevenson and Parsloe 1993).

Collective empowerment

At a broader level, opportunities for users and carers to have a voice in service planning include the preparation of community care plans, the drawing-up of service specifications and quality control. Such involvement is a way of ensuring that services will be relevant to users' needs, it recognizes the rights of users to a say in planning, it can promote greater efficiency in resource use and it increases organizations' public accountability (Connelly 1990; Croft and Beresford 1993).

In the case of community care plans, social services authorities have explored a variety of ways of enabling individual service users or user organizations to participate in the planning process. Consultation has typically involved public meetings, surveys, requests for information or focus groups (Hoyes *et al.* 1993; Bewley and Glendinning 1994). However, Bewley and Glendinning's study raised a number of questions about the extent to which users were able to influence the process: the agenda was frequently set beforehand, there was little time to consult more widely with other users and documents were often excessively long and used a good deal of jargon. User representatives might be chosen through personal invitation rather than through election or nomination by user organizations, and carers were selected instead of users (and not just in addition to them). While the study focused on the involvement of disabled people, it found that sensorily impaired people and members of black and other minority ethnic communities were often excluded. Users' support needs, in terms of additional training, transport and access to office services, were frequently unmet.

Similar issues arise in relation to user involvement in broader service planning. Users have drawn attention to tokenism, where one or two users are co-opted onto committees as a gesture of involvement, but with no real input into decision-making (Beresford and Campbell 1994). The difficulties facing user involvement are considerable; despite employing a number of methods to involve users and carers and obtain their views, many authorities have acknowledged that their initial efforts have been inadequate (Hoyes and Lart 1992). Part of the problem relates to practical difficulties in reaching a wide range of people. In addition, agencies often see users primarily as consumers; the focus of user involvement is then likely to be on consultation to obtain information about users' experiences of services and other services that may be required. Users will thus be expected to react to agencies' agendas, rather than being able to address the issues they themselves see as most important. Some users and user-led organizations feel such an approach does not allow them an adequate say in service planning. Their own wish is, rather, for greater participation in the planning process, in order to design services which more appropriately meet users' needs (Croft and Beresford 1990; Beresford and Campbell 1994). These different views about user involvement reflect the difference between the market and 'voice' models of empowerment: the model that is adopted will determine how much, and what kind of, say users have.

In work by the Office for Public Management (OPM), Goss and Miller

(1995) outlined a continuum of approaches to planning that are based on different working relationships between organizations and users (Box 3.3).

Box 3.3   A continuum of relationships between users, carers and staff in service planning and development

- No involvement
- Consumer education and 'marketing services'
- Limited two-way communication
- Listening and responsive
- Partnership

- *The closed model: no involvement.* In this approach, managers and professionals define the issues and problems. Any consultation is essentially cosmetic. No information is sought about users' views, professionals 'speak for' users, and decisions are made without reference to users.
- *Consumer education and 'marketing services'.* Again, this is based on managerial or professional definitions of the issues or problems. However, the approach uses market research to obtain users' views and gathers systematic data on users' needs. Aggregated information is used, in combination with managerial and professional expertise, to inform organizational decision-making.
- *Limited two-way communication: organization-centred listening.* While managers and professionals define the issues and problems, they use consultation procedures to obtain users' views. Support is provided to user groups. Users' views are collated, analysed and used to support decisions.
- *Listening and responsive.* Managers and professionals listen to users' descriptions of the issues and problems. Consultation is open-ended and a variety of forms of support is provided to user groups. This process enables the organization to gather ideas and suggestions about ways forward, which then form the basis for decisions. Users are involved in testing the success of subsequent actions.
- *Partnership.* Users, professionals and managers work together to identify issues and problems. There is open access and involvement of users at all stages of the planning process, with support to user groups. Problem-solving is 'user-led', and managers and users work together to identify possible solutions. Decisions are made jointly by the organization and users. Reviews and changes are also undertaken jointly.

The above framework is derived from a project involving users, carers and social services managers in a number of localities in England and Wales. An earlier study (Goss and Miller 1993) had noted the difficulties in involving users in planning: the failure to take full account of users' views, the lack of information for users, and a failure to adapt processes and timescales to meet users' needs and interests. There was also considerable confusion about the role that users could or should play. Authorities which superficially involved users reported relative satisfaction with their progress, while those with real commitment to engaging with users referred to the major problems they were encountering.

The OPM project focused on two major steps in the process of user involvement: establishing communication ('talking and hearing') and creating change in the way services are planned and managed. It identified a number of issues which needed to be addressed if greater user involvement were to be achieved: setting up new user networks, user involvement in the design of consultation processes, clarity of purpose, openness about the terms of reference, the provision of information in acceptable formats about services and planning procedures, timing of meetings, accessible venues, transport to meetings, money for administration costs, payments to users for advice or consultancy and the provision of training. Not least, agencies themselves must be prepared to make organizational and policy changes: at the moment, some well-meaning agencies appear to ask a good deal while offering little in return (Fiedler 1993; Goss and Miller 1995). These various issues provide a potential basis for evaluating the extent of user and carer empowerment in service planning.

Advocacy

Increasing calls for user involvement in decision-making at both an individual and a collective level have led to an increase in advocacy, self-advocacy and citizen advocacy schemes (cf. Butler and Forrest 1990; Campbell 1990; Morris 1993b; Bristol Advocacy Project 1993; Simons 1993; Webb and Holly 1994). The need for such advocacy arises from the limited amount of information often available to service users, and their lack of power in relation to professional staff and organizations that provide services. By helping people to make or express choices and to obtain the services they need, advocacy represents a means whereby people can gain or regain control over their own lives (Campbell 1990; Cale 1993). Even under the new community care arrangements, which are designed to give users a greater voice in services, users may still need support to ensure their needs are recognized and adequately met.

Advocacy includes both the development of skills on the part of individual service users, whereby they gain confidence to express their own feelings and wishes, and the voicing of collective concerns (Simons 1993). The form that advocacy schemes take varies according to the specific needs of particular user groups, the extent to which non-users are involved and the issues addressed. What they have in common, however, is a concern that users' views should be expressed and heard. The establishment of advocacy

schemes thus represents an important element in the process of empowerment. The extent to which their goals are achieved will reflect the outcomes
of that process.

Views about community care

General principles

Users' and carers' statements of what they want from community care
often reflect the principles that underpin *Caring for People*. Henwood *et
al.* (1993), for instance, reviewed four published accounts of users' views,
which generated 42 statements in three broad categories:

- the right to a normal pattern of life within the community;
- the right to be treated as an individual; and
- the right to additional help to develop maximum potential.

While their review was specifically of services for people with learning
disabilities, the principles and statements expressed by community care
service users and carers are often similar, even where specific needs may
be different (see Box 3.4).

**Box 3.4   Principles underpinning community care, as identified by users
and carers**

- Respect
- Autonomy
- Being treated as an individual
- Recognizing the totality of individual needs
- Choice
- Recognition of the work and needs of carers
- Partnership

Respect is based on the fact that users are both fellow human beings and
fellow citizens (Beeforth *et al.* 1990; Henwood *et al.* 1993; RADAR 1993;
South East Staffordshire District Joint Planning Group 1993). In relation
to service delivery, this includes a respect for users' privacy and dignity.
Respect is also needed for people's different racial, cultural and religious
backgrounds and values (Richardson *et al.* 1989; Wertheimer 1991; National Association of Race Equality Advisors 1992).

Autonomy involves the right to make decisions about one's own life.
Users may need practical help, but they must be able to determine what
form of help is provided (Morris 1993a). To view users as dependent is to
demean and devalue them.

Users and carers must be *treated as individuals*. They have individual needs and services must be sufficiently sensitive and flexible to respond to those needs (Jowell 1991; National Association of Race Equality Advisors 1992; Henwood *et al.* 1993). Users may, for instance, need practical assistance, while preferring personal care to be provided by family or friends (Morris 1993a).

People also have a *range of needs*, and a number of different forms of support may then be needed to assist people to lead full and independent lives. This includes independent living within their own homes and full participation in the life of the community and wider social networks (Beeforth *et al.* 1990; Centre for Policy on Ageing 1990; NCVO 1992; South East Staffordshire District Joint Planning Group 1993).

The need for *choice* applies to all aspects of service provision. It may, for instance, refer to the type of accommodation required or who people should live with (Henwood *et al.* 1993). Beeforth *et al.* (1990) call for a choice of alternatives to hospitalization for people with mental health problems; disabled people in Staffordshire have asserted their right to the social interactions they themselves choose and to the support they need to achieve these (ibid. 1993); carers want to be able to choose what care they are to provide (NCVO 1992); and disabled users of personal care services want choice about the timing of daily activities, such as when to get up or go to bed (Morris 1993a; RADAR 1993). All too often, though, choice is lacking. Allen *et al.* (1992) found that few older people had any choice about care provision: the only 'choice' available was usually negative – to refuse or discontinue a service.

Agencies have frequently failed to *recognize the work and needs of carers* (Carers' Alliance n.d.; Richardson *et al.* 1989). This has sometimes led to professionals imposing further burdens on carers, instead of relieving them (Wertheimer 1991). It is vital to take full account of the specific wishes of carers themselves and to tailor services to their individual needs and circumstances (Richardson *et al.* 1989). Older carers have voiced a specific plea for equity for all carers, regardless of their age (Alison and Wright 1990).

Not least, users and carers have called for *partnership* in decision-making about services in general (Carers' Alliance n.d.; Richardson *et al.* 1989; Henwood *et al.* 1993). This includes the identification of the services that are required. It also involves participation in the way services are managed and in their evaluation (Beeforth *et al.* 1990).

The scope of community care

A number of reports and statements by users note that their quality of life in the community is often dependent on many services other than those provided (or purchased) by the NHS and SSDs. Indeed, the lack of other services can have a far greater impact on their lives than those arranged by the NHS or SSDs: users and carers therefore stress the need to see 'community care' in its broadest sense (Wertheimer 1991). Comments have frequently been made about:

- the lack of an adequate income and the serious difficulties caused by poverty (Beeforth *et al.* 1990; Carers' Alliance n.d.; King's Fund 1988; Richardson *et al.* 1989; Wertheimer 1991; NCVO 1992; Robertson 1993; Rogers *et al.* 1993);
- poor housing, or even a total lack of it, which can aggravate both physical and psychological problems (Beeforth *et al.* 1990; Wertheimer 1991; NCVO 1992; Rogers *et al.* 1993);
- a lack of employment opportunities, or of support to obtain and retain employment (Beeforth *et al.* 1990; NCVO 1992; Henwood *et al.* 1993; Rogers *et al.* 1993);
- inadequate or expensive transport facilities, which prevent people from obtaining services or participating in community life (Wertheimer 1991).

The older people who spoke to Robertson (1993) made a distinction between basic needs (including warmth, good health care and an adequate income) and the needs and services that may be considered in relation to community care assessments. If basic needs are not being met, 'putting in help with meals, with shopping, with cleaning or with getting dressed etc. makes a mockery of care' (1993: 17).

Specific services needed from SSDs

Users have identified a wide range of services that either reflect gaps in current provision or whose availability is restricted. The responsibility for some of those services lies with SSDs; in other cases, it may be shared with other agencies:

- support with basic daily living, including self-care and meals (Alison and Wright 1990; Centre for Policy on Ageing 1990; Wyn Thomas 1990; Wertheimer 1991);
- practical help in the home, and regardless of any need for assistance with personal care (Morris 1993a; South East Staffordshire District Joint Planning Group 1993);
- suitable accommodation, both for families and for individuals (Alison and Wright 1990);
- use of a telephone (Alison and Wright 1990; RADAR 1993) – this has been identified as a basic need (Robertson 1993);
- special equipment and adaptations, provided on the basis of need, not SSDs' financial considerations (South East Staffordshire District Joint Planning Group 1993; Keep and Clarkson 1994);
- post-diagnosis advice and support for disabled people, their families and friends (South East Staffordshire District Joint Planning Group 1993);

- special transport facilities, where public transport is unavailable or unsuitable (Wertheimer 1991; RADAR 1993);
- support to use community facilities and engage in social activities (Henwood *et al.* 1993; Rogers *et al.* 1993);
- the opportunity for both users and carers to have holidays (Alison and Wright 1990; Henwood *et al.* 1993; NCVO 1992; RADAR 1993);
- day centres (West Suffolk Health Authority and Suffolk County Council 1992);
- support for carers, including practical help and the opportunity for short or longer breaks from caring (Carers' Alliance n.d.; Richardson *et al.* 1989; Alison and Wright 1990; Wyn Thomas 1990; London Research Centre 1991; NCVO 1992; West Suffolk Health Authority and Suffolk County Council 1992; South East Staffordshire District Joint Planning Group 1993);
- social work contact and support (Alison and Wright 1990; London Research Centre 1991);
- crisis intervention houses in the community for people with mental health problems (Beeforth *et al.* 1990; Rogers *et al.* 1993);
- physical access to buildings (South East Staffordshire District Joint Planning Group 1993);
- the opportunity to develop skills, including literacy and daily living activities (Henwood *et al.* 1993);
- emotional support, including befriending schemes, individual counselling, users' groups and carers' support groups (King's Fund 1988; Richardson *et al.* 1989; Beeforth *et al.* 1990; Centre for Policy on Ageing 1990; Wyn Thomas 1990; Rogers *et al.* 1993);
- advice about benefits (King's Fund 1988; Henwood *et al.* 1993; Robertson 1993; South East Staffordshire District Joint Planning Group 1993);
- support for people who have been discharged from hospital (Rogers *et al.* 1993);
- interpreter services for people whose first language is not English or who have sensory impairments (National Association of Race Equality Advisors 1992; South East Staffordshire District Joint Planning Group 1993);
- the support of an advocate (Beeforth *et al.* 1990; Henwood *et al.* 1993);
- the need for agencies to monitor people's general well-being and what happens to them (Beeforth *et al.* 1990);
- the need to improve public understanding of people's circumstances and needs, and to counter hostility and intolerance (Rogers *et al.* 1993).

Improving existing services

Both broad and more specific improvements need to be made to existing service provision in order to make it acceptable to users and carers. Problems arise from:

- a lack of information about the services available (King's Fund 1988; Richardson *et al.* 1989; Alison and Wright 1990; Beeforth *et al.* 1990; Wyn Thomas 1990; Jowell 1991; London Research Centre 1991; NCVO 1992; Robertson 1993; Henwood *et al.* 1993);
- the failure of SSDs to publicize the criteria by which they prioritize needs and services (RADAR 1993);
- incomprehensible information and use of jargon (Beeforth *et al.* 1990; Henwood *et al.* 1993);
- a complex and unclear community care system and procedures (Jowell 1991);
- delays in assessment and service provision – a frequent cause of complaints (Keep and Clarkson 1994);
- having to ask for services a long time in advance (Wertheimer 1991);
- prohibitive charges for home care, adaptations or respite care – leading to users and carers being unable to use services (South East Staffordshire District Joint Planning Group 1993; Keep and Clarkson 1994);
- a failure to allow users to determine how work is to be carried out (Morris 1993a).

Users and carers have also pointed out that the process of service delivery can be of value in its own right, quite apart from the content and more explicit objectives of the service itself. Older people, for example, have expressed their appreciation of the contact with volunteers who deliver meals on wheels (West Suffolk Health Authority and Suffolk County Council 1992). Elsewhere, the users of a community psychogeriatric service and their carers felt that practical help from health and social services made only a marginal difference to their lives: nevertheless, they attached considerable importance to the concern and caring attitude shown by staff (Wilson 1993).

Conclusions

While formidable enough as it stands, the above list of principles, services and problems does not seek to be comprehensive: it merely reflects some of the points made by users and carers in a small number of selected documents. Chapter 2 (p. 42) referred to the 178 outcome criteria identified by service users and providers in Trafford in relation to residential care for older people: comparable numbers of criteria could no doubt be drawn up for each of the many other community care services. The range of issues that could potentially be included in any evaluation of community care outcomes is thus extensive. Nor would it be limited to aspects of services themselves: account should arguably also be taken of specific short- and longer-term objectives that have been worked out with individual users and carers, and of the ways in which they could potentially be assisted to lead more fulfilling lives.

A number of the views outlined above pre-date the introduction of the new community care arrangements. Others overlap with the aims under-pinning those arrangements, as is the case, for instance, in respect of choice, partnership and autonomy. In any evaluation of community care, it is necessary to establish not only the extent to which users' and carers' specific service needs are met, but also whether broader objectives such as user involvement and empowerment have been achieved.

Some research has been carried out on the development of outcome measures based on users' and carers' expectations and on the concept of empowerment. Schalock *et al.* (1989), for instance, included aspects of choice in their work on the quality of life for people with learning disabilit-ies. Barnes (in Cormie and Crichton 1994) has developed a questionnaire to establish whether membership of user panels leads to increased empower-ment for older people. The questionnaire is designed to explore changes in panel members' self-esteem and control over their lives as a result of participation in the panels. Within the field of learning disability, the 'five accomplishments' model examines the extent to which service users are able to live an 'ordinary life': it includes the dimensions of choice, independ-ence, community presence, respect and community participation (O'Brien and Lyle 1987). However, service practitioners have found it hard to incorp-orate this model into routine practice (Henwood *et al.* 1993). The model also fails to take account of users' and professionals' potential disagreements about desirable objectives: not all users, for instance, wish to develop skills to increase their independence or achieve 'valued social roles'. Similarly, Stevenson and Parsloe (1993) point out that some people may feel over-whelmed, rather than empowered, by, say, participation in case conferences; older people may want an acknowledgement of their wish for dependency or the need to use savings to purchase services may be experienced as disempowering.

Research on empowerment needs to take account of users' and carers' own preferences: to be empowered, they must be able to express their feel-ings and needs, and feel they have some control over their lives. Broader measures of empowerment, common to all users of community care ser-vices, could include people's general awareness of entitlement to services and the ability to determine how and when a service is provided (Stevenson and Parsloe 1993). At the level of involvement in service planning, empower-ment would be reflected in users' and carers' ability to shape the agenda, exercise influence and make decisions.

Summary

The new community care arrangements place considerable emphasis on the greater involvement of users and carers in service planning. Official guidance indeed refers to their 'empowerment' and to the 'redressing of the balance of power' between users and carers on the one hand and agencies on the other. Such empowerment calls for a major change in the way individuals' needs are assessed and care packages designed, as well as in broader planning at an agency level. The new arrangements do, in theory, offer users and carers new opportunities to identify their needs and specify the services they require. However, if the success of those arrangements is to be adequately monitored, measures of empowerment need to be developed: such development is currently at a very early stage.

Just as user and carer involvement is a key feature of service planning, so outcome measurement should itself be informed by users' and carers' views about community care. Those views are underpinned by a number of general principles. Users and carers call for respect and to be treated as individuals. They want autonomy in deciding how to lead their lives and a choice in all aspects of the services that are provided to help them do so. Carers specifically seek a recognition, too often missing in the past, of the work they carry out and of their own needs. In addition, users and carers have detailed a wide range of community care services that they need, including both improvements to existing services and additional services. The variety of their needs presents a real challenge to the task of measuring outcomes.

Further reading

Beeforth, M., Conlan, E., Field, V., Hoser, B. and Sayce, L. (eds) (1990) *Whose Service is it Anyway?: users' views on co-ordinating community care*. London: Research and Development for Psychiatry (The Sainsbury Centre for Mental Health).
   Gives users' views about mental health services and the need for user involvement in service planning.
Goss, S. and Miller, C. (1995) *From Margin to Mainstream: developing user- and carer-centred community care*. York: Joseph Rowntree Foundation and Community Care.
   Reports on a series of projects designed to extend user and carer involvement in community care.
Henwood, M. with Vyvyan, C. and Renshaw, J. (1993) *Measuring Up To The Strategy? Learning Difficulties, Quality and the All Wales Strategy*. Cardiff: Welsh Office and Audit Commission.
   A survey of how quality of service provision for people with learning difficulties is being monitored in Wales. Compares checklists of quality criteria derived from policy sources and from users' views, and examines the extent to which existing instruments include those criteria.
Hoyes, L., Jeffers, S., Lart, R., Means, R. and Taylor, M. (1993) *User Empowerment and the Reform of Community Care*. Bristol: School for Advanced Urban Studies.

A study of the structures and processes for collectively involving users and carers in community care planning. Reviews background issues and local authorities' intentions.

Keep, J. and Clarkson, J. (1994) *Disabled People Have Rights: final report on a two-year project funded by the Nuffield Provincial Hospitals Trust*. London: The Royal Association for Disability and Rehabilitation.
Reports on 700 complaints made by disabled people about the provision of social services.

Morris, J. and Lindow, V. (1993) *User Participation in Community Care Services*. Leeds: Community Care Support Force, NHS Management Executive.
Suggests ways in which community care agencies can promote user choice and control in service provision, and user involvement in planning and purchasing.

Richardson, A., Unell, J. and Aston, B. (1989) *A New Deal for Carers*. London: King's Fund Centre.
Discusses carers' needs, describes practical ways of meeting those needs, and outlines policies that need to be adopted by service agencies.

Stevenson, O. and Parsloe, P. (1993) *Community Care and Empowerment*. York: Joseph Rowntree Foundation.
Discussion of the nature of empowerment in community care.

Turner, M. (1997) Reshaping our lives. *Research, Policy and Planning*, 15, 2: 23–25.
Description of a project designed to research the way in which service users and their organizations are defining and working towards the outcomes they want for themselves, and to develop well-researched and well-founded user perspectives on outcomes.

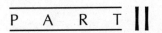

PART II

OUTCOME MEASUREMENT

CHAPTER 4

PEOPLE WITH PHYSICAL IMPAIRMENTS

Introduction

Community care services for people with physical impairments have received low priority in comparison with services for other user groups (Beardshaw 1988; Social Services Inspectorate/NHSME 1993a). In contrast to other users, people with physical impairments have not been the subject of major policy changes (such as the closure of long-stay institutions) which might have warranted research input to document people's needs or the impact of new policies. The majority of people with physical impairments are older people, and the impact of disability is frequently seen as one aspect of the experience of ageing. A concern with community care for older people has resulted from projected increases in the numbers of frail older people, together with a concern to develop non-residential support services for older people. There have not been any comparable policy imperatives to stimulate research into community care for the smaller number of people with physical impairments under retirement age.

Consequently, the measures that do exist have most frequently been developed in relation to rehabilitation, physiotherapy and occupational therapy services – some of these measures will be briefly reviewed here. Inherent in these services, however, is the concept of change in personal functioning. But while occupational therapy is an important component of social services provision, more clinical concerns essentially lie within the health care rather than the social care sector. The relevance of clinically-oriented measures to community care is therefore questionable.

Existing measures are of limited value for two further reasons (see Box 4.1). First, it is necessary to distinguish between clinical interventions aimed at treating medical problems and the objectives of social support services.

The aim of the latter is not the achievement of better health status, nor is it, in the main, to improve physical functioning. It involves, rather, the provision of support to enable people to lead independent lives – as is indeed emphasized in *Caring for People*. Secondly, a focus on physical functioning or health status reflects a 'medical' model of disability, in which disability is defined in terms of physical malfunctioning that requires medical intervention. The 'social' model, on the other hand, focuses on the attitudinal, institutional and environmental barriers that disabled people encounter within society; this reflects the context-dependent nature of disability. If disabled people are to lead independent lives, it is these barriers that need to be addressed – and appropriate outcome measures need to be designed.

Box 4.1   Limitations of existing measures

- Focus is on clinical interventions, rather than social support to assist people to lead independent lives
- They are generally based on a medical rather than social model of disability

---

An increasing general awareness of the social model and of the importance of independent living is largely due to disabled people's criticisms of professional attitudes and practices and their development of a framework for policy practice that is based on disabled people's own concerns. Many of those concerns are reflected in the new community care arrangements: the need for disabled people to have choice and control, to be able to decide what services are needed and to lead independent lives. At the same time, a number of disabled people feel that 'community care', in the way it has often been provided, militates against such principles. Morris (1993a), for instance, argues that a system based on residential care for frail older people typically fosters dependence: services have been provided for people who can demonstrate their helplessness, whereas what is needed is support for people who wish to increase – not decrease – their independence. Outcome measurement must accordingly focus not on the 'care' elements of community care services, but on the extent to which those services promote independence. As discussed later in this chapter, such concerns are beginning to inform research and evaluation, though work to develop appropriate outcome measures for routine use is still at a very early stage.

Measures used by professional staff

The measures that are currently available primarily reflect the concerns of professional staff. Measures have, for instance, been developed to describe initial functional status, monitor progress, allow comparisons between disabled people, illustrate degrees of independence or dependence, establish the effectiveness of clinical input and indicate what care and support services will be required (Jeffrey 1993). A large variety of measures is available, and there is a broad degree of agreement between them about the aspects to be investigated. However, there is often a lack of comparability between results obtained using different measures: a study of the relative sensitivity to change of four separate measures found that none of the instruments seemed consistently most sensitive (Fitzpatrick *et al.* 1992b). A review of the available measures has suggested there is no 'perfect' instrument available for general use, and a combination of instruments may be required (Fricke 1993). This is particularly true in the detailed investigation of specific disabilities, such as severe head injury (for example, Greenwood and McMillan 1993) or stroke (for example, Wolfe 1993). Here we will focus on some of the broader measures that are available.

McLellan (1992) suggests that the most important goals for rehabilitation services relate to self-care, communication, mobility, continence, fulfilling activities (especially employment), adequate finance and the needs of informal carers. The WHO's *International Classification of Impairments, Disabilities and Handicaps* (ICIDH) identifies six dimensions of the social impact of disability: orientation, physical independence, mobility, occupation, social integration, and economic self-sufficiency (World Health Organization 1980). In practice, the specific goals of rehabilitation depend on the skills and responsibilities of different professional groups. Occupational therapists, for instance, define rehabilitation as assisting people to regain function or to compensate for its loss, and they focus specifically on activities of daily living (Jeffrey 1993).

Two categories of existing measures will be considered here:

- Functional status measures that examine the ability to perform basic activities of daily living and the degree of loss of independence, for instance in relation to self-care and mobility. Such measures are frequently used by community occupational therapists or other rehabilitation staff to monitor the progress of treatment or to assess outcome (Charlton 1989).
- Comprehensive rehabilitation measures, including indices of general health status.

Examples of these, discussed below, are summarized in Box 4.2.

Functional status measures

Two of the functional status measures in most common use in community occupational therapy are the Barthel Index and the Functional Independence Measure (Fricke 1993; Jeffrey 1993).

Box 4.2   Examples of functional and health status measures

- Barthel Index
- Functional Independence Measure
- Sickness Impact Profile
- Functional Limitations Profile
- Nottingham Health Profile
- SF-36
- Rosser Disability and Distress Scale

The Barthel Index

The Barthel Index (BI) was designed to assess disabled people's degree of functional independence. It has been used to assess patients before admission to hospital and after discharge, patients who could benefit from rehabilitation programmes, predict length of stay, estimate prognosis, predict functioning at home, determine when to discharge people home, anticipate outcomes and evaluate services (McDowell and Newell 1987; Wilkin *et al.* 1992; Tennant *et al.* 1993).

The BI consists of ten items, each of which is rated according to whether the person is unable to perform the task, requires help or can manage independently. The ten items are:

Feeding	Mobility
Transfer from chair to bed	Climbing stairs
Personal hygiene	Dressing
Use of toilet	Control of bladder
Bathing	Control of bowels

Each item is scored as 0, 5, 10 and 15, with the highest scores indicating independence; scores are then summed to give a total from 0 to 100. The BI can be completed within a few minutes, and can therefore be incorporated relatively easily into routine practice. It does, however, require the assessor to have considerable knowledge of the individual's abilities and circumstances.

The BI's scoring system has been subject to criticism: changes indicated by a given number of points do not reflect equivalent changes in functional independence across different activities. There is also insufficient evidence of its responsiveness to change: substantial change can occur within the broad categories without altering index scores (Wilkin *et al.* 1992). The authors have noted that even a score of 100 does not necessarily mean that no help is required: the index focuses solely on self-care and does not, for example, include tasks of daily living such as cooking or shopping, nor does it take account of mental status or social well-being (Bowling 1991).

Some commentators have expressed reservations about the BI's lack of sensitivity at the independence end of the scale, the lack of clarity in some of the terminology (such as being able to complete tasks 'in a reasonable time'), the fact that the summed score effectively cancels out an improvement in one area if there is deterioration in another, its insensitivity to improved rehabilitation outcomes that do not result in changes in score and possible confusion in comparing results between different people (Eakin 1989a,b; Tennant *et al.* 1993). Bowling (1991) concludes that its simplicity poses severe limitations and cannot, therefore, recommend its use. However, others have described it as an appropriate measure to demonstrate the proportion of people who gain independence and to compare different rehabilitation programmes, especially in relation to the more severe functional difficulties found in rehabilitation work and in the care of older people (Fitzpatrick *et al.* 1992b; Tennant *et al.* 1993). Some health authorities are using the BI in joint assessment programmes with SSDs, to determine whether people need nursing home care.

The Functional Independence Measure

The need for a specific measure for physical rehabilitation resulted in the creation of the Functional Independence Measure (FIM). This is a 19-item rating scale that covers self-care skills, mobility, communication, cognitive ability and social adjustment – representing four of the WHO's six categories as compared with the BI's two (McDowell and Newell 1987; Jeffrey 1993). It has been used in a number of studies, and a comparison study of the FIM and BI is currently being carried out in West Lothian (Jeffrey 1993).

Comprehensive rehabilitation measures and health status indices

These measures have two underlying features (Jeffrey 1993):

- a holistic approach to function, examining the broad quality of life of disabled people and their carers; and
- a concern with disabled people's own views of desirable outcomes rather than a focus on professionals' objectives.

The Sickness Impact Profile and Functional Limitations Profile

The Sickness Impact Profile (SIP) measures the perceived impact of sickness on people's daily activities. It consists of 136 statements in 12 categories:

Sleep and rest	Mobility
Eating	Body care and movement
Work	Social interaction
Home management	Alertness behaviour
Recreation and pastimes	Emotional behaviour
Ambulation	Communication

Respondents are asked to describe their actual behaviour on a given day by giving 'yes' answers, where appropriate, to the specified statements. Weights were produced for the relative severity of limitation implied by each statement and scores can be summed up for individual categories, for the instrument as a whole, and across two dimensions: physical and psychosocial.

While the SIP was developed in the USA, the Functional Limitations Profile (FLP) is a version of the SIP that was adapted for use in the UK. The measures can be self-completed or administered by an interviewer, taking 20–30 minutes to complete (McDowell and Newell 1987). The SIP has been found to be especially useful in studies of people with chronic illness (Wilkin *et al.* 1992). The FLP has also been used to assess change over time within the same individuals (Fitzpatrick *et al.* 1992b). While it has proved sensitive to such change, the authors caution that interpretation must take account of the particular measurement properties of the instrument (Fitzpatrick *et al.* 1992b); preliminary findings from another study indicate that contextual information is needed in order to explain causality. The length of the measures means they are perhaps more suited to research rather than operational purposes. However, one of the authors of the FLP has noted that not all its aspects will be relevant in every case in which it is used (Charlton 1989).

The Nottingham Health Profile

The Nottingham Health Profile (NHP) is a self-completion questionnaire that examines aspects of people's perceived physical health, emotional well-being and social functioning. It is similar to the SIP in its focus on the impact of disease on the individual. Unlike the SIP, though, it asks about feelings and emotional states directly, rather than examining behavioural consequences (McDowell and Newell 1987).

The NHP consists of two parts. The first includes 38 statements, grouped into six sections:

Physical mobility	Energy
Pain	Sleep disturbance
Emotional reactions	Social isolation

Respondents are asked to indicate whether they experience the problems described in the 38 statements. Scores are summed up within each section, using a weighting system for the individual items, but there is no overall score for the measure as a whole. The second part of the NHP, which can be used independently of the first, asks about the effect of the person's state of health on activity in seven areas of everyday life:

Paid employment   Sex life
Household tasks   Interests and hobbies
Social life   Holidays
Family relationships

However, the developers of the scale subsequently suggested that this part
should not be used until further developmental work had been completed
(Bowling 1991).

The NHP is widely used and has the advantage of brevity: the first part
can be completed in less than 10 minutes. It is seen as being more suited
to people with severe problems or chronic illness than to those with minor
health problems (Wilkin *et al.* 1992). However, a number of problems have
been identified. The yes/no answers, for example, are insufficiently sensitive for some respondents (Wilkin *et al.* 1992). Answers are supposed to
reflect problems 'at the moment', but this may be interpreted differently by
different people. Its brevity means that it cannot be a comprehensive measure of quality of life. Bowling (1991: 64) comments that it provides only
a 'shallow' profile of functional difficulties, psychological disturbance and
social functioning, while some problems (such as sensory difficulties, incontinence or eating problems) are not assessed at all. Despite the fact that
pain is one of its six dimensions, weaknesses have been reported in distinguishing, for example, migraine sufferers from the general population
(Wilkin *et al.* 1992). While it has been tested for its ability to discriminate
between different groups of people, Bowling (1991) suggests that, because
it focuses on more severe health problems, minor improvements over time
are unlikely to be detected.

The Short Form 36 health survey questionnaire

The Short Form 36 (SF-36) health survey questionnaire is a general measure of health outcome. It is a self-completion instrument that takes 5–10
minutes to complete. Bowling (1995) notes that it is fast becoming one of
the most frequently used health status measures.

The SF-36 examines three aspects of health: functional status, well-being
and 'overall evaluation of health'. These are measured by 36 questions,
grouped into eight categories:

Physical functioning
Social functioning
Role limitations due to physical problems
Role limitations due to emotional problems
Mental health
Energy and vitality
Pain
General perceptions of health

In six of these categories, respondents are asked to rate their responses on three- or six-point scales. Scores are summed up within the eight categories.

The SF-36 is shorter than the SIP and has been shown to overcome the NHP's inability to detect low levels of difficulties (Brazier *et al.* 1992). Further work is being carried out to test its sensitivity to changes in individuals' health (Garratt *et al.* 1993). However, the physical functioning scale has been criticized for focusing too much on mobility and not taking sufficient account of potential changes in domestic skill levels (Anderson *et al.* 1993). The general nature of the questions also means that the SF-36 cannot, on its own, provide a full assessment of people's potential difficulties: a more specific functional scale would need to be used as well (Jenkinson *et al.* 1993; Bowling 1995).

The Rosser Disability and Distress Scale

Unlike the NHP, FLP and SF-36, the Rosser scale was designed for completion by clinical staff, although a version for self-completion has been proposed. It has been used as a general measure of health output, as a basis for calculating Quality Adjusted Life Years (QALYs) and to inform policy decisions (Wilkin *et al.* 1992).

The scale is made up of eight levels of functional difficulty and four degrees of distress. It can be completed in 10 seconds, though staff may need to draw on other sources of information such as observation or a separate assessment – for which a questionnaire has been produced (Williams 1988). While Rosser herself has produced a scaling system on the basis of the views of a number of professionals and laypeople, alternative valuations would be possible. Once a valuation system has been chosen, the results can be summed up into a single score.

As it stands, the distress category incorporates a number of different and potentially conflicting dimensions, such as physical pain and emotional distress, but further developmental work is taking place on this. The scale has been recommended for use where a quality of life measure is required but where longer health profiles would be unsuitable for repeated application (Rawles *et al.* 1992). Others have suggested, though, that it might most appropriately be used in conjunction with disease-specific or more comprehensive general measures, as a means of setting findings in a wider context (Wilkin *et al.* 1992). It is also seen as likely to play an increasingly important role in resource allocation (Wilkin *et al.* 1992).

An approach based on a social model of disability

While existing outcome measures focus largely on rehabilitation or health, other concerns will often underpin the provision of community care services for people with physical impairments. Disabled people in Derbyshire, for instance, have identified seven key areas of need (Silburn 1993): information – to enable choices to be made; counselling – to help make those choices; housing which is suitable, accessible and well-located; technical aids or enabling equipment; personal assistance when it is needed; transport – to function in society; access – to all public buildings and amenities. Some of these issues were highlighted in a report on community care for younger disabled people, carried out by the Social Services Inspectorate and NHS Management Executive (Social Services Inspectorate/NHSME 1993a). This report noted that housing, personal support, opportunities for jobs, education and leisure pursuits, access and transport are all vital components of a comprehensive community care service for disabled people. In a research study into the transition to adulthood, Hirst and Baldwin (1994) used a structured questionnaire to examine young disabled people's experiences of independent living, employment, financial independence, self-esteem, a sense of personal control, spare-time activities and friendships. The young people saw these aspects as fundamental to leading 'a normal life'.

Measuring outcomes

Work by the Massachusetts Interagency Council on Independent Living (ICIL) in the early 1980s sought to translate two of these issues – living arrangements and productivity (including contributions to family and community life) – into rating scales to measure independent living outcomes (De Jong 1981). The ICIL model ranked seven living arrangement outcomes and 12 productivity outcomes on a scale of 0 to 10; information was also gathered about people's marital status, age, sex, the severity and duration of the impairment, environmental variables such as transportation barriers and economic disincentives. An initial study of people with spinal cord injuries involved the use of six research instruments, including a mailed and an interview questionnaire.

De Jong noted that the study represented only a beginning for future research on independent living issues. In a review of this study, Parmenter (1988) suggested that a more comprehensive approach should include domains such as: control over one's life, meaningful participation in decision-making processes, the development of an adequate self-image and satisfaction with one's lifestyle. Parmenter himself proposed a model for the quality of life of people with physical impairments which included 37 domains in three broad categories:

- individuals' perception of self, including cognitive and affective dimensions and aspects of personal lifestyle;
- individuals' behaviours in relation to social interaction, occupational and material well-being, accommodation and access to services and facilities;
- societal influences.

The model is based on a 'symbolic interactionist/ecological' theoretical framework and makes clear that the quality of life of disabled people is dependent on the environment in which they live. In operationalizing this model, Parmenter includes elements of individual functioning, the broader environment and relationships between the two. Although his approach adopts a broader societal focus, the inclusion of individual functioning suggests the continuing influence of the medical model, which members of the disability movement might not find acceptable. However, the domains in his model do provide further indications of aspects that might be included in more systematic outcome measurement for disabled people.

Basing outcome measurement on the views of disabled people

The social model itself arose as a reaction to the professional dominance of services for disabled people and to the medical model on which those services were based. The measures reviewed earlier in this chapter reflect the medical model. However, both disabled people and – as has been noted – *Caring for People* have called for a reorientation of community care services to a model where service users have 'a greater say in how they live their lives and the services they need to help them to do so' (para 1.8). The same principle applies to outcome measurement. It is not enough that measures should be said to be 'acceptable' to disabled people on the basis that questions are easy to answer or that questionnaires have been completed. Rather, outcome measurement must be based on disabled people's own views of the important issues: other approaches are likely to be inappropriate. An approach based on a social model of disability should consider the points outlined in Box 4.3.

Box 4.3   An approach based on a social model of disability

- Take account of the full range of disabled people's needs
- Focus on the societal and environmental issues that affect individuals, not on individual impairments
- Use disabled people's own definitions of need

An increasing number of projects are now seeking to develop services that are more appropriate and more responsive to disabled people. User participation in service development is, for instance, a central tenet of the projects initiated by the Living Options Partnership at the King's Fund Centre (Fiedler and Twitchin 1992; Fiedler 1993). The standards against which effective services and good practice might be evaluated include (Fiedler 1991):

- the extent to which services meet users' needs, expectations and preferences;
- the opportunity for disabled people to exercise real power over the way services and policies are planned and implemented; and
- partnership between users and service providers.

The Partnership also identified 33 aspects of a good service system, such as a choice of housing options, opportunities to experience increased independence and appropriate personal assistance to facilitate independent living (Fiedler 1991). A subsequent report examined evaluation in the context of user involvement in the commissioning of services (Morris 1995). It stressed that the success of services should be measured in terms of their effectiveness in improving the quality of users' lives. The specific measures to be used would depend on the service being evaluated. Attention would also need to be paid to the varying needs and experiences of people with different impairments: those impairments can be static or progressive, and can be acquired at different stages in life (Morris 1995). Some implications for research include the points in Box 4.4.

Box 4.4   Implications for research

- Focus needs to be on the effectiveness of services in improving the quality of people's lives. This will involve objectives such as:

  independent living
  the choice of appropriate housing
  availability of appropriate personal assistance
  a voice in determining the type of services to be provided
- Disabled people must be fully involved in the research

Some research studies have begun to examine aspects of outcomes for disabled people, using the social model. A study of personal assistance schemes, for instance, included questions about choice and control, and specifically control over the type of assistance provided, how it is provided, the times at which it is provided, and by whom (Zarb and Nadash 1994). Research currently under way at the Policy Studies Institute, in association with the Disability Research Unit at the University of Leeds, is examining the inclusion and exclusion of disabled people in the social, political and economic lives of their communities (Zarb et al. 1994). An important part of this study is to develop ways of measuring the participation of individual disabled people in decisions about community support services. The views and involvement of disabled people are key features of the study. Only through such involvement can outcome measures be developed which reflect the extent to which community care policies are meeting disabled people's needs.

Conclusions

This chapter has considered some of the measures that have been used in relation to services for people with physical impairments. Most of the existing measures focus on aspects of rehabilitation or health; they also tend to be driven by professional or clinical concerns and are based on a medical model of disability. Such measures do not address the objectives of community care; they also conflict with the emphasis on user involvement and empowerment within the new community care arrangements. If, moreover, the purpose of services is to enable people to lead a normal life, it can be argued that outcomes should not be based on changes in measured states. Rather, the examination of outcomes should take account of the extent to which people have to change their lifestyles because of a lack of appropriate services.

No methods currently exist to address comprehensively the outcomes of community care for people with physical impairments. However, this chapter has outlined some of the service developments that are taking place which are based on a social model of disability and which seek to make services more responsive to disabled people's needs. The principles underpinning such services – such as independent living, a choice of services, control over the services provided, and user involvement in service planning – provide a potential framework for the evaluation of their outcomes.

Summary

Outcome measurement for people with physical impairments has most frequently been carried out in relation to rehabilitation or occupational therapy services. While a number of measures have been designed in these and other clinical contexts, many relate to specific physical conditions or problems.

The more general measures fall into two main categories. Functional status measures focus on the ability to perform basic activities of daily living and on the extent of functional independence. Such measures include the Barthel Index and the Functional Independence Measure, both of which have been designed for completion by professional staff. More comprehensive rehabilitation measures include indices of general health status: examples of these are the Functional Limitations Profile, Nottingham Health Profile and SF-36. The focus of such measures, however, is on rehabilitation and health. These measures also tend to be based on a medical model of disability, in which disability is defined in terms of physical malfunctioning that requires medical intervention, thus reinforcing a perception of disabled people as objects of medical attention. The medical model has been heavily criticized by many disabled people. They advocate, instead, a social model that focuses on the barriers that disabled people encounter within society, thus reflecting the context-dependent nature of disability.

A new approach to outcome measurement is needed in relation to the provision of social support services, where objectives may include the promotion of independent living, choice of appropriate housing, availability of appropriate personal assistance, and a voice in determining what services are required. Some work has been carried out on measuring aspects of living arrangements, employment, choice and control. However, further work is needed to develop appropriate methods of assessing the effectiveness of services in improving the quality of disabled people's lives. Fundamental to any such work is the need to involve disabled people in deciding what is to be measured, and how.

Further reading

Fiedler, B. (1991) *Tracking Success: testing services for people with severe physical and sensory disabilities.* Project Paper No. 2, Living Options in Practice. London: King's Fund Centre.

Sets out a range of criteria for assessing whether effective services are available, based on standards in six key areas: a response point to users' needs, a place to live, personal support services, access to the community, specialist services, and opportunities for personal development.

Morris, (1993) *Independent Lives? Community Care and Disabled People.* Basingstoke: Macmillan.

Discusses the nature of independent living and describes the experiences of disabled people living in the community. Argues that community care can reduce, rather than enhance, disabled people's ability to lead independent lives.

Morris, J. (1995) *The Power to Change. Commissioning Health and Social Services with Disabled People.* Partnership Paper No. 2, Living Options Partnership, London: King's Fund Centre.

Discusses outcome measurement within the context of disabled people's involvement in the commissioning of health and social services. Notes that outcome measurement should be based on disabled people's experiences of services, and describes how users can be involved in setting standards against which to measure outcomes.

CHAPTER 5

OLDER PEOPLE

Introduction

Most older people come into the orbit of the community care system as a consequence of health-related problems. It is perhaps not surprising, then, that many of the measures currently used relate to physical and mental health and physical functioning. Community care services have been aimed at rehabilitation or, more frequently, at the prevention of admission to residential care. There are numerous schedules and scales available for assessing older people (see, for example, Kane and Kane 1981; Israel *et al.* 1984; Thompson 1995). In particular, there is a proliferation of scales to assess different aspects of psychological functioning. However, when standardized scales have been used in the social care field, they have mainly sought to assess need rather than outcome. In recent years there have been some attempts to evaluate the outcome of community services for older people, although, as might be expected, these have concentrated on groups of particular policy interest such as people on the margin of need for residential care (Challis and Davies 1986; Knapp *et al.* 1992) and people with dementia (Gilleard 1987; Levin *et al.* 1989).

The main domains used in studies of outcome for older people come broadly under the headings of functional capacity, mental state, morale, social functioning and level of service provision (Box 5.1). Rates of mortality and institutionalization are also often cited as outcome measures. Studies which look at outcomes for carers of older people tend to focus on their health and levels of burden or stress, and these will be considered in greater detail in Chapter 8. Here each of the main domains is considered in turn, to see which instruments have commonly been used in work with older people.

Box 5.1   Domains measured in studies involving older people

- Functional capacity – physical and cognitive functioning
- Mental state – depression, anxiety
- Morale – subjective well-being
- Social functioning – integration, engagement
- Service provision (an intermediate outcome)

Measurement domains

Functional capacity

A variety of instruments has been used by researchers to assess changes in the functional capacity of older people. Perhaps the best known measure of these is the Katz Activities of Daily Living (ADL) Index. This comprises six basic activities:

Bathing	Transfer
Dressing	Continence
Toileting	Feeding

The Index was used by Challis and Davies (1986) in conjunction with a composite measure of general health based on a screening schedule developed by Bergmann *et al.* (1975) which covered eyesight, hearing, breathlessness, giddiness, risk of falling, incontinence and a self-assessment. Outcome was defined as the change occurring between assessments at two points in time.

Another well-known instrument is the Clifton Assessment Procedures for the Elderly (CAPE). This instrument includes a Behaviour Rating Schedule (BRS) that examines four dimensions (Pattie and Gilleard 1979):

Physical disability	Communication difficulties
Apathy	Social disturbance

The BRS was used by Knapp *et al.* (1992) to assess changes in behaviour and skills within the *Care in the Community* demonstration projects for older people.

In two studies undertaken by the Research Team for Care of the Elderly at the University of Wales College of Medicine, functional capacity was assessed using an ADL index described by Townsend (1979), in which respondents assess their ability to perform nine everyday tasks. One of the studies was concerned with the effect of health visitors working with older patients in general practice (Vetter *et al.* 1984); the other examined outcomes for older people three months after discharge from hospital (Victor and Vetter 1989).

A study of older people by Neill and Williams (1992) also focused on those who were discharged from hospital to community care. The researchers used a six-item Guttman scale which had previously been used by, among others, Arber *et al.* (1988). In addition, respondents were asked about their ability to perform 18 self-care tasks, using a list which had been developed and used by the National Institute for Social Work Research Unit (Social Services Inspectorate 1990c). The study found that the 18 items were particularly sensitive to change in respect of very old and frail people, most of whom had high dependency ratings according to the Guttman scale.

Finally, Askham and Thompson (1990) used performance tests of daily tasks when evaluating a home support scheme for older people with dementia, because of the difficulty in using measures based on self-report with this group of people. The tests were based on a modified version of the Performance of Activities of Daily Living Scale or PADL (Kuriansky *et al.* 1976).

Mental state

A variety of assessment instruments have also been used in studies which have looked at outcomes for older people in terms of changes in depressed mood. For example, Challis and Davis (1986) used the 12-item General Health Questionnaire (Goldberg 1972), whereas the Depression Inventory of Snaith *et al.* (1971) was used in the evaluation of both the social care scheme in Gateshead (Challis *et al.* 1990) and the *Care in the Community* demonstration projects (Knapp *et al.* 1992). Vetter *et al.* (1984) studied the impact of health visiting and examined anxiety and depression using a scale developed by Foulds and Bedford (1979). The Geriatric Mental State (GMS) schedule (Copeland *et al.* 1976) was used by Levin *et al.* (1985, 1989) to assess changes in the mental state of the older people in their study; in this case, the schedule was completed by a research psychiatrist.

Neill and Williams' (1992) study of hospital discharge used the Self-care (D), as developed by Bird *et al.* (1987), to assess for depressed mood two weeks and three months after discharge. Askham and Thompson (1990) assessed changes over time in the mental state in older people with dementia in the home support scheme, using two scales from the Comprehensive Assessment and Referral Examination (CARE) Schedule (Gurland 1980): the CARE Organic Brain Syndrome scale and the CARE Depression scale (from which the Self-care (D) is derived).

Davies and Challis' (1986) evaluation of the Kent Community Care scheme included an assessment of older people's organic mental state, using nine items developed by Bergman *et al.* (1975), but these were not used to measure outcomes. A randomized controlled trial of a community support scheme for older patients discharged from hospital (Townsend *et al.* 1988) used a mental test score (Denham and Jeffreys 1972) to assess cognitive function. However, in the research studies that have assessed social care outcomes for older people in terms of mental state, more attention has generally been paid, understandably perhaps, to the detection of changes in depressed mood and anxiety rather than in cognitive functioning.

Where older people suffer from dementia, it may be important to be aware of changes in their levels of cognitive functioning. Although it is unlikely that community care services will be directed towards attempting to secure improvements in this area, ways may need to be found to deal with potential deterioration as the disease progresses. Ramsay *et al.* (1995) reviewed existing standardized assessment instruments as possible community care outcome measures for people with dementia, but found that few of them had all of a range of characteristics deemed to be desirable in such measures. Those characteristics included both technical requirements (outlined in Box 5.2) and requirements which were designed to ensure ease of administration, such as: taking less than 30 minutes to complete; being in a format that was suitable for routine practice; being suitable for use by different professional staff; and not being restricted to institutional settings.

Box 5.2   Technical criteria for potential outcome measures

- Validity   content covers important domains, is consistent with other measures, discriminates between different groups
- Reliability   produces the same results if repeated, or used by a different observer
- Responsiveness   sufficiently sensitive to detect changes

Ramsay *et al.* (1995) identified some possible measures, all of which would need further testing or development. The possibility of obtaining subjective views from people with dementia was not considered. This latter issue represents a new area for research and development: although some relevant work is currently taking place, most studies of people with dementia rely on professional assessments and the opinions of informal carers.

Morale

This assessment domain covers subjective well-being, including life satisfaction and self-esteem. Of all the domains, this is the one where there is least variation in the instruments used to assess outcomes for older people. Studies by Challis and Davies (1986), Challis *et al.* (1990), Knapp *et al.* (1992) and Townsend *et al.* (1988) all used an anglicized 17-item version (Challis and Knapp 1980) of the Philadelphia Geriatric Centre (PGC) morale scale developed by Lawton (1975). In a recent review of quality of life instruments for everyday use with older patients (Fletcher *et al.* 1992), the anglicized version of the PGC morale scale was the leading contender for routine clinical use and was the scale recommended by the Royal College of Physicians (1992) Joint Working Party with the British Geriatrics Society.

An alternative morale scale is the Southampton Self-esteem Scale (SES). This is based on a Dutch scale and was used to assess changes in self-esteem arising from living in an experimental sheltered housing scheme as an alternative to institutionalization (Coleman 1984). However, it has not, to date, been widely used and there is little evidence of its responsiveness to change (Fletcher *et al.* 1992).

Service provision

Changes in service provision have been used in some studies as a measure of outcome. In the terminology developed earlier in this book, such changes are intermediate rather than final outcomes, since the connection between changed service use and impact on the user cannot be assumed. Changes in service provision tend to be measured by means of a few questions developed for a particular study rather than by using a standardized scale. Outcome measures relating to service provision include: care shortfalls (Challis and Davies 1986); use of medical and social services (Vetter *et al.* 1984; Townsend *et al.* 1988); changes in home help provision (Neill and Williams 1992); and meeting the need for help (Davies *et al.* 1990).

Social functioning

This is a complex, conceptually confused area covering notions of social engagement, integration, social support and networks. It is perhaps not surprising, then, that measures of social functioning have been used less frequently as domains for outcome measurement than measures of functional capacity and mental state. Some of the few studies which have assessed social functioning in terms of outcomes for older people include Knapp *et al.* (1992), who used the Interview Schedule for Social Interaction (ISSI) (Henderson *et al.* 1980) and Challis and Davies (1986), who used a measure of social contact based on a count of weekly contacts (Tunstall 1966). Vetter *et al.* (1984) also included a few questions about the frequency of social contacts.

Outcome measures for older people

It is 15 years since Challis (1981) argued that the measurement of outcome in social care for older people was in its infancy, and there appears to be little evidence to suggest that we have moved much further forward since then. In relation to health care, there has been a belief at national level that some standardization of the assessment of older people would be useful (Royal College of Physicians 1992). To this end, the Royal College of Physicians ran joint workshops with the British Geriatrics Society to identify and recommend schedules and scales for assessing activities of daily living, communication (including hearing and vision), cognitive function, mood, morale and social status, with the hope that these assessments would be incorporated into standard clinical practice.

At the joint workshops, 'experts' reviewed the available scales for each assessment domain in turn. It is not clear from the report what criteria were used to draw up the shortlists for each domain. A small working group was established for each of the domains to consider a shortlist of scales, with reference to their validity, reliability, ease of use, sensitivity and responsiveness to change. The following scales were the recommended ones in the report:

- *Activities of daily living*: the Barthel Index (BI). A ten-item scale of primary ADL, as discussed in Chapter 4.
- *Communication*: the Lambeth Communication Scale (LCS). Four questions taken from the Lambeth Disability Screening Questionnaire asking about difficulties in seeing newsprint, recognizing people across the road, hearing a conversation and speaking.
- *Cognitive function*: the Abbreviated Mental Test Score (AMT). Ten items covering age, time, year, name of place, recognition of two persons, birthday, date of World War I, Queen's name, counting 20 to 1 backwards, five-minute recall, full street address.
- *Depression*: the Geriatric Depression Scale (GDS). A 30-item self-completion scale with yes/no answers relating to respondents' feelings over the past week. A shorter 15-question version is also available but was not recommended until further evaluation work has been carried out. Examples of questions include: 'Are you basically satisfied with your life?' and 'Do you often get bored?'
- *Morale*: the Philadelphia Geriatric Centre Morale Scale (PGCMS). A 17-item self-completion questionnaire relating to subjective well-being including questions such as 'Do you feel lonely much?' and 'Do you get upset easily?'

A standardized scale for assessing social status was not recommended; instead, a checklist of major social indicators was suggested, which might trigger the need for a fuller social assessment.

The instruments were recommended for use in geriatric hospital medicine, while also being seen as potentially appropriate for primary health care. However, the Barthel Index in particular is most suited to people with moderate to severe functional difficulties (Wilkin *et al.* 1992) and would be less relevant in social care and community settings where sensitivity and responsiveness to change are also required in relation to people with lower levels of difficulty.

A recent national survey of the assessments of older people by community nurses indicated that, while there was a considerable amount of structured assessment being undertaken, nurses were using a wide range of assessment instruments, including many which had been developed locally (Philp and Dunleavey 1994). Only three assessment instruments were currently widely used (that is, in more than 20 district health authorities): the Barthel Index (used in 33 per cent of DHAs); the Roper, Logan and Tierney nursing assessment instrument (in 19 per cent of DHAs); and the CAPE (in 18 per cent). There is clearly a potential for outcome measurement if the administration of these scales is repeated over time. Unfortunately, the authors were unable to access similar information about assessment activities in SSDs.

Measuring outcomes in routine practice

Within an acute hospital setting, an action research project has sought to assess the feasibility, costs and effectiveness of incorporating the above recommended instruments into routine practice (Philp *et al.* 1994). At first, it was envisaged that Senior House Officers (SHOs), as well as paramedical and social work staff, might contribute to the assessments. In practice, however, it was the nursing staff who conducted all the assessments with the exception of the AMT, this being administered by SHOs on admission (as had always been the case prior to the project). Only the nursing staff proved able to change their practice to undertake the new assessments. The researchers found that staff attitudes were generally positive; they understood the objectives of the scheme; it was easy to administer; it provided useful feedback and was generally perceived to improve the quality of patient care. Staff were less sure about whether they had been adequately involved in setting up the scheme or whether it had improved resource management. The information proved costly to collect in terms of staff time although the schedules were in addition to routine nursing documentation and the authors suggested that there would be some scope for reducing costs by integration of the assessment procedures. It is of interest that senior staff in this secondary care setting were particularly enthusiastic about the value of the post-discharge assessment, which the researchers had decided should be conducted. In addition, all staff rated the Relatives Stress Scale (another measure added by the researchers) more highly than the recommended scales in relation to its perceived usefulness, effects on decisions taken and increased knowledge about patients. Even in an acute setting, therefore, more detailed knowledge about social aspects of care was valued: this would suggest that, where the focus is more specifically on non-clinical aspects of community care, the recommended set of meas-ures may not be the most appropriate.

Other researchers have demonstrated, in work in two clinical settings, that it is feasible to collect routine outcome information (Parker *et al.* 1994). On both a geriatric assessment and rehabilitation unit and in a geriatric day hospital, the Barthel Index was administered. While it was capable of detecting change in older hospital in-patients, it was not appropriate for use with day hospital patients because of the 'ceiling effect' resulting from the high scores of most of the day patients. It would appear that the improve-ment of physical functioning may not be a suitable objective in relation to day care.

Professional and user views about service aims and objectives

It is clearly important that outcome measures should reflect the aims and objectives of the particular services to be evaluated. Older people them-selves appear to have had little input into determining assessment domains or the outcomes to be evaluated, despite calls for anti-ageist approaches (Hughes 1995) and empowerment-oriented practice (Cox and Parsons 1994). An interesting attempt was made by Roberts *et al.* (1994) to establish performance (or outcome) measures for geriatric medical services. They sought to obtain a consensus view from consultant geriatricians in three health regions and then asked geriatric day hospital patients for their views on the appropriateness and importance of the measures selected by the geriatricians. Both geriatricians and patients said the two most important performance measures were 'reducing disability' and 'improving quality of life', although the geriatricians placed the latter first while patients gave priority to 'reducing disability'. Both groups gave 'reducing mortality' low priority. Patients' third most important measure was 'reducing carer bur-den' (seventh out of twelve items on the geriatricians' list), while the geri-atricians placed more weight on 'effective medical treatment', 'consumer satisfaction' and 'problem resolution' than did the patients. Service users clearly place a high value on positive outcomes for carers. While it may be that cases in which there is conflict are of most concern to professionals, in many instances users and carers attach a great deal of importance to each other's welfare. Although this study was valuable in attempting to establish outcome measures for geriatric medical services, it did start very much from a consultant perspective, with user views being sought (in far fewer numbers) 'to balance professional opinion' (Roberts *et al.* 1994).

Questioning the use of standardized instruments

It has been argued that it is important to assess needs and outcomes for older people in the context of their individual biographies (Dant *et al.*

1989). In their evaluation of the Gloucester Care for Elderly People at Home Project, the researchers rejected the use of standardized measures, preferring to focus instead on the extent to which identified needs were met. The project involved three care coordinators, each of whom was attached to a primary health care team. Their role included negotiating with older people and reaching an agreement as to what their needs were and how they should be met. The researchers used, as their indicator of outcome, the extent to which these agreed needs were met. They then looked at the types of needs that had been identified and grouped them into six categories. These were based around:

- help that the care coordinator could provide, such as counselling, advice (such as about benefits), and simple aids to daily living that she was able to deliver;
- housing and the home;
- the person and their physical and mental state;
- activities of daily living and managing in the home;
- contact with statutory services; and
- contact with informal care.

Other commentators, too, have argued strongly against structured standardized assessment forms. Kemp and Middleton (1993), for instance, reject them because they are not user-focused or sufficiently related to individual needs and aspirations. Hill and Harries (1993), reflecting on their experience of administering the Short Form-36, identify some of the technical and methodological problems in using it as an outcome assessment instrument with older people. While they acknowledge that there is a role for structured outcome measures, they conclude that structured questionnaires largely reflect the opinions of 'experts', and that much might be gained from using less-structured techniques and listening to what older people have to say.

Conclusions

As has been noted, research studies have looked at outcomes for older people in terms of functional capacity, mental state, morale, level of service provision and social functioning with little attention being paid to user views and issues such as participation, choice and empowerment. As with people from learning difficulties, there can be problems eliciting the views of very frail older people and people suffering from dementia. However, many older people are able to give their views and these do not always coincide with the views of professionals. Much more work needs to be done in discovering the outcomes which are important to them.

There is evidence to suggest that structured assessments are being used by a large number of community health agencies, although a wide range of instruments is currently in use. It remains to be seen to what extent the instruments recommended by the Royal College of Physicians (1992) will be incorporated into routine clinical practice. In any case, it is as yet uncertain whether these or other measures will be suitable for use to assess outcomes in practice. At present we do not have a similarly detailed picture for SSDs: we do not know which, if any, standardized instruments are being used around the country for assessment, nor is there any recommended standard set of measures, or systematic approaches, which would reflect the objectives of personal social services in their work with older people. In neither health nor social care does it appear that repeated assessments are used to measure outcomes.

In a report aimed at social work practitioners, Hughes (1993) proposed a framework for the comprehensive assessment of older people and their carers. She also suggested ways in which assessments might be conducted and information collected *with* older people to foster user participation and empowerment. However, the measurement of outcomes for older people is not aided by the lack of a model of 'normal' or 'successful' ageing, and the absence of a professional consensus as to what constitutes a good quality of life for older people (Hughes 1990).

Summary

The prevention of permanent admission to residential care has long been an avowed objective of services for older people. Research-based studies of outcome in community care for older people have concentrated on more disabled groups, such as those with dementia, or those on the margin of need for residential care. Therefore, outcome indicators such as mortality and admission to residential care or hospital have been prominent; nevertheless, studies have also looked at functional capacity, psychological well-being and social functioning. Structured instruments are least well developed in the latter domain. Given that carers' attitudes are predictive of admission, these too have been a focus of interest. Ideas about normal lifestyles in old age have not yet been influential in relation to outcome measurement, although there is a stream of argument which reflects a lack of confidence in standardized methods and argues for a less structured and more individualized investigation of the extent to which people's needs have been met.

There has been considerable professional activity, both nationally and locally, in relation to attempts to introduce some consistency into the assessment of older people. Of course this may not always be relevant to the question of outcome, since not all assessment instruments reflect areas in which it is hoped to achieve change. Mental or physical ill-health have been important factors in bringing older people to the attention of community care services and this, coupled with the aim of avoiding residential care, perhaps explains the focus in assessment, on instruments which measure the capacity to manage activities of daily living, communication, mental state and levels of cognitive functioning. The influence of older people on the design of outcome measures or the specification of relevant domains appears to be minimal. Most measures reflect normative professional judgements about areas which are important influences on the likelihood of continuing at home, rather than factors which have been identified as contributing to quality of life (although some may have this effect as well).

Further reading

Bowling, A. (1995) *Measuring Disease*, pp. 278–281. Buckingham: Open University Press.
    Discusses assessment batteries (sets of measures) thought appropriate for older people. Many of the disease-specific measures in the book are clearly appropriate to older as well as younger people.
Bowling, A. (1991) *Measuring Health*. Buckingham: Open University Press.
    Chapter 6 discusses the measurement of social networks and social support.
Bowling, A. (1997) *Measuring Health*, 2nd edn. Buckingham: Open University Press.
Challis, D. and Davies, B. (1986) *Case Management in Community Care*. Aldershot: Gower Press.
    A study which measured and compared the outcomes, and costs, of contrasting forms of service provision for older people.
Ramsay, M., Winget, C. and Higginson, I. (1995) Review: Measures to determine the outcome of community services for people with dementia. *Age and Ageing*, 24: 78–83.
    Reviews measures used for assessment of people with dementia to determine their suitability in outcomes measures.

CHAPTER 6

PEOPLE WITH MENTAL HEALTH PROBLEMS

Introduction

A large number of scales are available for the measurement of outcomes in mental health services. These are extensively reviewed by Bowling (1995), who groups them into three categories: symptom scales, quality of life instruments, and role functioning and related instruments. Although most of these measures have been developed in health care settings, a number of the issues they examine are also relevant to social care: this reflects the fact that mental health problems have broad effects on people's lives and are often caused or aggravated by social, interpersonal or other contextual factors.

As was outlined in Chapter 1, the emphasis here will be on measuring the impact or effectiveness of services for individual users, not on administrative indicators of outcome such as prevalence, hospital admissions or re-admissions (Knapp *et al.* 1992). While an administrative approach can provide broad population and service-based data, it cannot reflect the full range of benefits (or possible failures) of services for users: for this, more specific measures of outcomes for individuals are needed.

An important issue in measuring individual outcomes is the extent to which objectives reflect the variety of individual circumstances and needs, or whether a more systematic or standardized approach is adopted. The production of individual care plans, for instance, offers a means of identifying both short- and long-term goals, and outcome measurement is then based on goal attainment. However, the individual focus of care plans means it may not be possible to make a precise comparison between outcomes for different users. On the other hand, the advantage of such an approach is precisely that it can take full account of the different mental health problems, needs, individual characteristics and circumstances of individual users: such factors militate against the use of more standardized methods. It is the care plan approach which underpins an outcome evaluation project carried out by the Health Services Management Centre in Birmingham (Green 1992). In this case, the focus is on the extent to which specific goals have been achieved for individual users, rather than on the production of aggregated data.

The main focus in this chapter, however, will be on the use of more systematic measures. A detailed review of a large number of measures is already available (Bowling 1995). The intention here will be to provide an overview of some of the measures that have been used in relation to community care or related fields, and to suggest some issues that need to be addressed in selecting or developing measures for use in routine practice situations.

The relocation of long-stay hospital patients into the community

A number of research projects have examined the impact of relocation policies on former long-stay hospital patients. The measurement instruments used in four of those projects will be considered here, together with the domains they covered; a summary of the broad categories of domains is shown in Box 6.1. A description of the four sets of instruments will be followed by some general comments about their applicability to outcome measurement in community care.

Box 6.1   Mental health: Examples of areas covered by existing measures

- Symptomatology and behaviour problems
- Social contacts and activities
- Morale and life satisfaction
- Everyday living skills

The Team for the Assessment of Psychiatric Services (TAPS) used a seven-part assessment schedule for long-stay patients moving out of Friern and Claybury Hospitals (O'Driscoll and Leff 1993). The authors noted that the most important area to assess was the well-being of the patients themselves. Their schedule accordingly consisted of the following:

- An original schedule for recording personal data and psychiatric history.
- An original index for establishing physical health.
- The Present State Examination (PSE), designed to establish the extent of

clinical mental health problems. (This superseded the initial use of the Krawiecka scale which was inappropriate for people who did not speak English or were otherwise unable or unwilling to provide information.)

- An original Social Behaviour Schedule, based on Wing's Ward Behaviour Schedule: this includes 'deficits of normal behaviour, such as poor self-care, and the presence of disturbed behaviour, such as verbal and physical hostility'. Information relating to the previous month is obtained from a member of staff.
- An original Patient Attitude Questionnaire, designed to elicit users' views about the services offered. After some initial questions to establish cognitive function, it asks for users' views about their current accommodation and service provision, and about possible future alternatives.
- An original Environmental Index, based on the Hospital Hostel Practices Profile (HHPP). The index seeks the views of professional staff about the environment in which users live, including the degree of autonomy they are able to exercise and the number of choices they can make.
- An original Social Network Schedule, which aims to establish, through interviews with users, the quantity and quality of social contacts over the previous month.

During the course of the project a further measure was developed:

- Basic Everyday Living Skills, used by staff to assess skills such as self-care, domestic skills and use of public amenities. Staff are also asked to assess the opportunities for independence available to individual patients.

Finally, a follow-up assessment (a year after people had left hospital) additionally included:

- A Community Services Receipt Schedule (developed in conjunction with the Personal Social Services Research Unit (PSSRU) at Kent University): this records services received in the community, unmet needs, and the principal carer's satisfaction with the quality and availability of each service.

The authors state that the package as a whole represents a compromise between a comprehensive and a manageable tool, given the several hundred patients requiring both initial and follow-up assessments.

The PSSRU's own evaluation of 28 *Care in the Community* pilot projects included eight mental health projects (Knapp *et al.* 1992). Their outcome dimensions covered: the type of accommodation provided; integration and opportunities; choice and empowerment; skills; symptoms and behaviour problems; social contacts; activities and engagement; morale and life satisfaction; and personal presentation. In order to assess these dimensions, they used the following instruments:

- A skills scale, incorporating items from the Social Behaviour Scale, Disability Assessment Schedule and Wykes's Social Performance Scale. This reflected the objective of both hospital and community-based rehabilitation training programmes to achieve skills in basic activities of daily living: cooking, housework, shopping, handling money, use of public transport, and looking after clothes and possessions.
- A scale to gather information about symptomatology and behavioural problems. Use of an instrument such as the PSE or other direct interviewer rating was excluded on the grounds that it would require more substantial resources. Instead, information was obtained from a staff member about 26 aspects of symptoms or behaviour.
- Questions on satisfaction with services.
- The Schedule for Social Interaction, to examine the extent of social contacts and activities.
- A battery of six instruments to assess morale and life satisfaction, including the Schedule for Social Interaction, a subscale of the Psychosocial Functioning Inventory, Seltzer and Seltzer's satisfaction questionnaire, Cantrill's Ladder (to assess general life satisfaction), and a depression inventory.
- A Client Service Receipt Interview (for community services).
- Information about personal presentation.

Unlike the above two projects, the Health Services Research Unit in North Wales mainly used existing instruments for its evaluation of patients discharged from the North Wales Hospital (Crosby and Barry 1995). Assessments were carried out at three-monthly intervals while patients were in hospital, as well as six weeks after discharge, after six months and after one year. Three main categories of outcome were measured:

- Mental state, using the Brief Psychiatric Rating Scale (BPRS), the Krawiecka Rating Scale and the Scale for the Assessment of Negative Symptoms.
- Social and behavioural functioning, using the Rehabilitation Evaluation of Hall and Baker (REHAB): this has sections on both deviant and general behaviour.
- Quality of life, with an instrument adapted from the model of Lehman *et al.* (1982). The revised schedule covers both objective and subjective evaluations in the domains of living situation, family relations, social relations, leisure activities, work, finances, religion, safety and health; additional questions concerned general life satisfaction. The schedule generally took 30–40 minutes to complete (Barry *et al.* 1992).

In addition, the HHPP was used to evaluate the flexibility and client-centredness of care arrangements, and a Staff Attitudes and Management Practices Schedule was designed to give further data on care practices.

In Northern Ireland, the Health and Health Care Research Unit worked in conjunction with PSSRU and the Unit for Research and Development for Psychiatry (RDP, now the Sainsbury Centre for Mental Health) to monitor and evaluate a *Care in the Community* programme (Donnelly *et al.* 1994). The same measures were used both for people with mental health problems and for those with learning disabilities. A baseline profile was obtained using a Community Placement Questionnaire, prepared by RDP, though with additional items from PSSRU's work on the Social Performance Schedule. The questionnaire, which was completed by staff, recorded both demographic data and assessments of factors that might affect placement, such as social functioning, problem behaviour, physical impairment and social contacts.

Prior to discharge, further measures were used to provide more detailed patient profiles and self-perceived quality of life:

- A Social Functioning Questionnaire, designed by RDP to assess a person's ability to perform basic activities of daily living related to self-care skills, domestic skills, social skills and responsibility. The inclusion of this measure within the earlier Community Placement Questionnaire enabled comparisons to be made between different points in time.
- A Problems Questionnaire (designed by RDP), containing items found on maladaptive behaviour scales.
- The PSSRU residents' interview, to measure morale and life satisfaction (as described above).

These three measures were repeated six months after discharge, after one year and after two years.

The above studies represent a detailed evaluation of the needs of former long-stay hospital patients and of the outcomes of their relocation in the community. Despite the comments about limited resources or having to adopt a 'compromise' approach, they required considerably more time and a much greater input of resources than would be available to service agencies in the course of their everyday work. The availability of those resources did, nonetheless, enable them to use or design a range of instruments to measure a wide variety of domains that together comprise community living.

Three general points must be made about the applicability of these studies to outcome measurement in community care (Box 6.2). First, the focus was on people who had, in many cases, been hospitalized for a number of years. One of the main objectives of the research was to measure what changes resulted from their move back into the community, but the baseline reflected their skill levels and general functioning within a long-stay hospital setting. While not denying that the same domains might need to be considered in respect of other people with mental health problems, the relative importance of particular issues and the appropriateness of specific measures would need to be reassessed if they were to be used in a different context.

Box 6.2　Measures used in relocation research

- Baseline is long-stay hospital rather than community living
- Designed by clinicians or researchers
- Too wide-ranging for use in routine practice

Secondly, the measures were designed by clinicians or researchers on the basis of their own perceptions of the relevant issues, and were frequently completed by staff members. Certainly users were sometimes asked for their views about the services provided or those they required. However, it is important in relation to routine practice in community care that users' views should inform the outcome measurement process, and that measures should include objectives such as the extent of autonomy, choice or independence they are able to exercise. At the same time, we recognize that the nature of mental health problems means that it is sometimes considered necessary to overrule individuals' own views or wishes in the interests of their own wellbeing or that of other people. The specific outcome measures to be used will thus need to take account of such considerations.

Thirdly, the studies illustrate the wide range of aspects of community living and services that can be included in the evaluation of mental health outcomes. The instruments are both detailed and take a considerable amount of time to complete, and it is far from clear whether or how they might be adapted for more routine use.

Examples of measures for routine use are being developed for the community mental health services. Given the overlap between health and social services in this field, some of those measures may be relevant to social care. We will now consider the area of overlap between health and social care, and some of the measures that span these two areas, and then describe a number of approaches to the development of outcome measures for routine use.

Outcome measurement in community psychiatric care

Clinical research uses

The outcome measures used in studies of community mental health services depend on both the purpose of the study and the resources available. Burns *et al.* (1993), for example, examined clinical and social outcomes in both a traditional and a home-based acute psychiatric service. A researcher

was available to carry out assessments within two weeks of the initial clinical contact, and at six weeks, six months and twelve months. The study
used a total of ten assessment schedules, of which the last four were for
completion with relatives or close friends:

- an initial social history;
- the PSE, to examine current mental state;
- the BPRS, to measure change in psychotic disorders;
- a clinical interview;
- the Social Functioning Schedule (SFS), covering social functioning in 12
  areas: employment, household chores, contribution to the household,
  money, self-care, marital relationship, care of children, patient–child
  relationships, patient–parent and household relationships, social contacts, hobbies and spare-time activities;
- a 37-item consumer satisfaction scale, which examined the quality, appropriateness and accessibility of care;
- the Family Burden Scale, measuring objective and subjective burden and
  subjective stress;
- 18 BPRS items, used to obtain a relative's or friend's assessment of
  symptoms;
- a relative's or friend's assessment of social functioning;
- a relative's or friend's satisfaction scale.

Service monitoring

Other approaches have been developed for more regular use. Shanks and
Gillen (1992) report on a project to identify simple measures of outcome
that would be suitable for general clinical use. The primary focus of this
study was on aggregated data rather than individual clinical information.
It involved the use of a small number of existing measures that were brief
and easy to use:

- The Global Assessment of Functioning scale (GAF), completed by clinical
  staff to assess symptomatology and functioning. The scale takes around
  5 minutes to complete.
- The General Well-Being Index (GWBI), designed to enable patients to
  indicate their level of well-being. During the course of the study, the
  index was replaced by the 28-item General Health Questionnaire (GHQ-
  28). The GHQ-28 can be completed in 3–4 minutes.
- The GHQ-28, used to obtain the self-rating of carers or 'significant
  others'.

The GHQ is essentially a screening instrument, designed to establish the
presence of non-psychotic illness or affective disorder. While Wilkin *et al.*
(1992) feel that evidence is lacking about its responsiveness to clinically

significant change, Bowling (1991) notes that it has been used to compare ratings at different points in time. In Shanks and Gillen's study, assessments were carried out with a random sample of patients within two weeks of initial contact and after six months. For patients who were discharged from care, the second assessment took place prior to discharge. The authors state that their method provides a useful basis for obtaining the views of users and carers, and the measures themselves are simple to use. They suggest that it could, with modest additional resources, be used on an intermittent regular basis.

Routine clinical use

Other work focuses on outcome measurement instruments that would be appropriate for routine clinical use. Five examples of such work will be described here.

Psychiatric Research in Service Measurement (PRISM): Institute of Psychiatry

Work currently in progress in Camberwell is using a four-measure package to assess needs and outcomes:

- The Camberwell Assessment of Need. This covers a range of 22 topics including, for example, accommodation, self-care, psychological distress and intimate relationships. Both users and staff are asked to record whether there is currently a problem in each of the topic areas, help received from informal carers or from paid staff and help required. There is space under each topic for an action plan.
- The GAF, used to examine clinical and social functioning.
- The BPRS.
- A version for patients of the Verona Service Satisfaction Scale, an 87-item questionnaire for completion by users.

Health of the Nation Outcome Scales (HoNOS): Royal College of Psychiatrists Research Unit

The publication of the White Paper *The Health of the Nation* highlighted the need for outcome scales to monitor the target of 'improving significantly the health and social functioning of mentally ill people'. Draft scales were accordingly prepared in 1992 and were subsequently revised and piloted; further trials took place in 1994 and a final report was due in 1995.

The aim of HoNOS is to provide a measure that is short enough to be used on repeated occasions as a routine component of Care Programme reviews. The data can also be aggregated to indicate overall changes in health and social functioning in the population as a whole. Its authors state that a portfolio of currently available instruments would be 'impossibly long and tedious to complete in routine clinical work' (RCP n.d.: 6). HoNOS itself consists (in its 4th version) of 12 problem areas relating to behavioural problems, impairment of personal functioning, symptoms of mental disorder, and interpersonal and social problems (RCP 1995) (Box 6.3). Each area is rated on a five-point scale to indicate the severity of problems. In the first pilot phase, involving a longer form, completion initially took 15–30 minutes: completion of the revised form is expected to require just a couple of minutes during routine use. A separate form for users to complete is comparable to the clinical one; a form for carers was also being prepared.

Box 6.3   Items in the HoNOS scales (4th version) (all are rated on a scale of 0–4)

 1 Overactive, aggressive, disruptive behaviour
 2 Non-accidental self-injury
 3 Problem drinking or drug-taking
 4 Cognitive problems
 5 Physical illness or disability problems
 6 Problems associated with hallucinations and delusions
 7 Problems with depressed mood
 8 Other mental or behaviour problems
 9 Problems with relationships
10 Problems with activities of daily living
11 Problems with living conditions
12 Problems with occupation and activities

The HoNOS forms were revised in the light of experience during piloting, and many pilot sites reportedly found them useful as a way of measuring outcomes. Nevertheless, one site stated that they were of limited use for confused older people: clinical progress may often be hard to achieve with this group of users, and the forms do not take sufficient account of the benefits and positive work that may nonetheless be taking place. This site suggested that the forms were more helpful as an epidemiological than as a clinical tool. Such comments may not be representative of all the pilot sites: others reportedly value the opportunity to gather and use standardized data, and further reports are awaited. Although four of the 12 problem areas are concerned with social aspects (relationships; activities of daily living; living conditions; and occupation and activities), additional information is likely to be required for the broader assessment of community care outcomes.

The FACE Outcomes Project: Quality Development Unit, Royal College of Psychiatrists

The aim of the FACE outcomes project is to develop a computerized outcome system for mental health services that can be used as part of routine clinical practice. The system is designed to measure the severity of problems and service outcomes; it includes the capacity to record data on service provision and aims to be acceptable to staff working in both health and social services. Development work began in 1990 and final implementation was due in 1995.

The FACE framework is based on six major axes:

Mental health	Social circumstances
Personal functioning	Physical health
Interpersonal relationships	Informal carers

Each axis has a number of levels. 'Personal functioning', for example, is broken down into areas such as self-care, domestic activities and community living skills; the authors suggest that this is the level at which an initial assessment might be made. At the next level, self-care is broken down into sets of specific problems related to, for instance, washing, shaving or dressing: it is at this level that a primary care nurse might conduct an assessment or monitor progress.

Global rating system used by Berger et al.

Both PRISM and FACE aim to incorporate outcome measurement into routine clinical work; to do this, though, complex data systems are required. In contrast, Berger et al. (1993) describe an approach to outcome evaluation in child and adolescent mental health services which synthesizes the key aspects of outcomes into a brief data-set. Their approach takes account of the heterogeneity of clients and problems, the views of different stakeholders and moderating factors that lie outside clinical control.

In addition to basic information about individual characteristics, clinical symptoms, interventions and number of contacts, the data-set includes nine questions about moderating factors and global ratings. The moderating factors include problem characteristics (complexity and severity) and case manageability (compliance and the controllability of external factors). The global ratings indicate clinical change, outcome in relation to the referrer's aims, and the patient's, carers' and referrer's perceptions of outcome. Each question is accompanied by a four- to seven-item scale. While the approach lacks the detail of other measures, it has the advantages of brevity and simplicity and provides global outcome ratings. On the other hand, the authors recognize that in-depth outcome studies would be needed to examine the details of each of the scales.

Case Management Project: Research and Development in Psychiatry (now the Sainsbury Centre for Mental Health)

The RDP project involved the development of case management in a number of pilot sites, and subsequent monitoring using a computerized database (RDP 1992). A total of 39 assessment and outcome indicators covered ten domains:

Physical health	Home supports
Mental health	Daily living skills
Medication	Occupation and daytime activity
Finance	Social network
Housing	Legal issues

The documentation also included a personal plan (incorporating users' own long-term goals) and records of contacts with staff. The system allowed for an overall evaluation of effectiveness in relation to symptomatology, quality of life, social support and social functioning. The importance given to non-clinical issues certainly reflected the broader aspects of daily living that are the concern of community care services. Although it involved additional record-keeping, it provided a means of monitoring the effectiveness of the service provided.

Quality of life

While the concept of 'quality of life' is potentially relevant to all users of community care services, much research and developmental work has taken place in the context of mental health service provision. Lehman *et al.* (1982), for example, examined eight aspects of the lives of people with chronic mental health problems: living situation, family relations, social relations, leisure activities, work, finances, safety and health (Box 6.4). Although their work was based on earlier studies of psychiatric patients and general quality of life work, they felt that definitive criteria for quality of life remained elusive. Their method has nonetheless provided a basis for other work, such as that of the Health Services Research Unit, described above.

Box 6.4   Dimensions of quality of life

• Living situation	• Work
• Family relations	• Finances
• Social relations	• Safety
• Leisure activities	• Health

Quality of Life Index for Mental Health (QLI-MH)

Becker *et al.* (1993) argue that most existing instruments, including that of Lehman *et al.*, have serious limitations. In the first place, patient input into their design was often minimal or non-existent. Secondly, the lack of consensus about domain content means that equal weighting for all domains, or even unequal but pre-set weighting, may not reflect the importance ascribed to them by individuals. Their own Quality of Life Index for Mental Health is based on existing scales but covers a range of objective and subjective, generic and specific domains. It was developed in the USA in conjunction with patients, family members and mental health professionals and is intended for use in routine practice.

The QLI-MH takes a three-dimensional approach involving: the measurement of nine domains by the patient, service provider and family at different points in time. The domains are:

Satisfaction   Finances
Occupational activities   Activities of daily living
Psychological well-being   Symptoms
Physical health   Goal attainment
Social relations

Information about patients' values is obtained by weighting each domain according to the patient's evaluation of its importance: this is seen as one of the strengths of the index (Bowling 1995). Questionnaires can be completed by service providers in 10–20 minutes, and by patients in 20–30 minutes, though assistance is sometimes necessary. Bowling (1995) suggests that, although further testing is needed of the QLI-MH's psychometric properties, it could prove to be a popular quality of life measure.

Lancashire Quality of Life (QOL) Profile

While the QLI-MH is intended for use in clinical settings, the Lancashire Quality of Life Profile was designed for use by either social or health care agencies (Oliver 1991). Testing took place in a variety of settings, including community mental health centres, but its main pilot phase consisted of over 400 interviews with clients of Lancashire SSD. The profile is based on existing research instruments, principally the model of Lehman *et al.* It is, however, intended for standard operational use, including both routine management monitoring and the evaluation of individual clients' progress (Mental Health Social Work Research and Development Unit 1993).

The QOL Profile includes nine domains:

Work or education   Finances
Leisure and participation   Living circumstances
Religion   Legal and safety issues

Family relations   Health
Social relations

In addition to yes/no questions, each domain includes questions which are answered with a seven-point Life Satisfaction Scale. Two other sections include questions about self-concept and a Cantrill's Ladder to indicate general well-being. Finally, the interviewer uses a uniscale (ranging from 'lowest quality' to 'highest quality') to mark their own rating of the person's present quality of life. The questionnaire takes an average of 37 minutes to complete.

The label 'quality of life' does not indicate a narrower focus than that of more comprehensive approaches. In terms of the domains included, the profile differs from the RDP model, for example, only in its exclusion of clinical questions about symptomatology and medication. However, a further difference is that, while administered by an interviewer, information is mainly gathered directly from service users (apart from the final uniscale).

The QOL Profile was not tested as an outcome measure. Nevertheless, Oliver (1991) suggests that the outcomes of human services relate to users' life conditions and that the profile might be used for the continued monitoring and review of users' general health and welfare. The broad scope of the profile, though, extends beyond the more specific issues that community care services may seek to address – even though those issues will vary for different individuals. The usefulness of the profile as a potential outcome measure then depends on whether a broad picture is sought about a person's quality of life or whether the focus is on the outcomes of specific services.

A question also has to be raised about the extent to which the QOL Profile incorporates the concerns and values of users themselves. Although the model used by Lehman *et al.* was designed to explore users' perceptions of their lives, the items for both that model and for the profile appear to have been drawn up by professionals. Oliver notes that 'very few clients ... complained about the interview'. However, some of the questions may be perceived as intrusive or irrelevant to the purpose of the interview, for example details of income, family composition or religion. The overall focus of the profile is also on individuals themselves, with the implicit suggestion that difficulties reflect something about the individual rather than the nature of the world around them. Finally, the profile does not address issues such as choice, empowerment or autonomy, all of which are central features of the current community care arrangements.

Satisfaction

The problems associated with measuring satisfaction were discussed in Chapter 2. Nevertheless, a number of measures of satisfaction have been developed in relation to health services in general. In the case of mental health services, the General Satisfaction Questionnaire (GSQ) is an example of a measure that was specifically designed for service evaluation in the UK (Huxley and Mohamad 1991). Based on users' own experiences, the GSQ is a short questionnaire that is available in different formats depending on the specific service context in which it is used (for instance, day centres or community support services). It has four main dimensions:

- a global measure of satisfaction;
- the user's view of service effectiveness;
- the accessibility of the service; and
- the acceptability of the service.

While the questionnaire does examine some of the more specific aspects of individual services, a distinction must nonetheless be drawn between a user's satisfaction with a service and the benefits that the service may or may not be providing in terms of desirable outcomes.

Conclusions

Many of the measures described in this section have been designed for use in clinical settings. While their more specifically clinical dimensions may not be directly relevant to outcome measurement in social care services, measures relating to social functioning or quality of life may appropriately be used in a social care setting. The Lancashire QOL Profile, for instance, was designed for use in either a health or social care context. However, its broad scope, length, professional orientation and lack of direct association with the objectives of community care suggest that considerable work would be necessary if it were to inform the development of routine outcome measures. A completely different approach is suggested by the global rating system of Berger et al. While this model could be adapted for use in community care, its brevity is achieved at the expense of any real detail about specific outcomes for individual users.

In a review of the mental illness specific grant, the SSI noted that a number of projects sought to promote principles such as those that underpin the NHS and Community Care Act: independence, choice and personal control (Social Services Inspectorate 1993b) (Box 6.5). It is such dimensions that need to be incorporated into any evaluation of the outcomes of community care. Of the measures reviewed above, only some of the work on deinstitutionalization formally sought to examine issues such as choice – for instance, in relation to how people spent their time and the activities they undertook (for example Knapp et al. 1992). The challenge now will be to establish how these dimensions of community care can be included in measures for more routine use.

Box 6.5   **Principles underpinning community care**

- Independence
- Choice
- Personal control

Summary

A large number of scales are available for the measurement of outcomes in mental health services. While they have often been developed for use in health care settings, some of the issues they examine (such as social functioning or quality of care) may also be relevant to outcome measurement within social care services.

Given the wide range of factors that can contribute to mental health problems, or be affected by service provision, many studies have used a battery of measures to ensure that a number of potentially relevant issues are covered. Detailed assessments and reviews may be an accepted part of medical or nursing practice. Although the introduction of care management and formal assessment procedures in social care again involves the detailed consideration of needs, it is unclear whether the routine use of lengthy measures would be as acceptable to social care practitioners or to service users as it is to psychiatric staff. On the other hand, brevity is generally only achieved at the expense of detail, while a more open-ended approach will fail to provide systematic comparative data about outcomes for different service users.

Another feature of most existing measures for use in health care settings is the apparent lack of user involvement in identifying the relevant issues or designing appropriate instruments. In addition, many of them rely on the provision of information by professional staff rather than on self-completion by service users themselves.

Of the work on mental health outcomes in social rather than health care, most has been concerned with the relocation of patients from long-stay psychiatric hospitals. Such work has involved the use of existing or new research instruments to examine a variety of aspects of people's lives. Even the shorter packages of measures have included a range of issues, such as mental state, social and behavioural functioning, and quality of life – and they have taken a good deal of time to complete. While such measures indicate the variety of domains that together comprise community living, their overall length rules them out for routine use by Social Services Departments. In addition, measures designed to examine outcomes for former long-stay patients may not be appropriate for a community-based population.

An alternative approach has involved the development of a quality of life instrument, such as was used in a variety of mental health service settings by one Social Services Department. This measure, however, is also long and broad-ranging and it did not involve users or carers in its development. Nor does it specifically address some of the fundamental objectives of community care (as outlined by the SSI): independence, choice and personal control. There remains a need to incorporate such objectives into measures that can be used in routine practice.

Further reading

A range of measures and approaches have been designed for use in different contexts. While the following references are relevant to the development of measures in community care contexts, they do not reflect the full range of measures available.

Green, S. (1992) *Measuring Outcomes in the Mental Health Services*. Discussion Paper 29. Birmingham: Health Services Management Centre, University of Birmingham.
Describes a project to measure outcomes for people with mental health problems in a hospital setting. The identification of the problems faced by individuals provided the basis for outcome evaluation.

Knapp, M., Cambridge, P., Thomason, C., Beecham, J., Allen, C. and Darton, R. (1992) *Care in the Community: challenge and demonstration*. Canterbury: Personal Social Services Research Unit, University of Kent.
Evaluation of 28 *Care in the Community* pilot projects for people being discharged from long-stay hospitals, including eight mental health projects. Used a range of outcome measures to examine social integration, choice and empowerment, skills development, symptoms and behaviour problems, involvement in activities, morale and life satisfaction, and personal presentation.

Oliver, J., Huxley, P., Bridges, K. and Mohamad, H. (1996) *Quality of Life and Mental Health Services*. London: Routledge.
A comprehensive introduction to the Lancashire Quality of Life Profile and its use in service evaluation.

RCP (1995) *Health of the Nation Outcome Scales: Version 4*. London: Royal College of Psychiatrists Research Unit.
Describes the fourth version of the HoNOS outcome scales, designed for use in mental health services. Consists of ten scales, each focusing on one area of a person's possible problems or lifestyle. Includes background notes to assist completion.

CHAPTER 7

PEOPLE WITH LEARNING DISABILITIES

Introduction

Ideas about the achievement of an ordinary life, and the importance of assisting people to undertake socially valued roles, have probably been more influential in relation to people with learning disabilities than any other group of service users. For adults, research-based measurement of outcome has most frequently taken place in situations where people have been discharged from long-stay hospitals, and in many ways the principles which reflect widely accepted objectives for services are the inferred opposites of institutional practice. Most frequently measured are competence and behaviour, community presence and participation, engagement in meaningful activity and individual morale or satisfaction. Experience in this field demonstrates that an established set of principles with wide support does not automatically give agreement on what constitutes correct practice: there may still be disagreement about acceptable levels of risk-taking, or about how actively staff should intervene to change people's behaviour, for example. Within such debates, it can be difficult to give the voice of the service user the prominence that might be wished. As will be outlined, there are a range of difficulties in ascertaining the views of people with learning disabilities, only some of which may be tackled by the use and development of appropriate techniques of communication.

Although it is accepted that characteristics of the living environment may be considered an external, or non-subjective, reflection of an individual's quality of life, there will be no detailed consideration of service evaluation techniques which take a systems approach, and thereby measure quality of care environments rather than outcomes for individuals. These measures have been comprehensively reviewed elsewhere (Raynes 1988).

Outcome measurement

Much outcome measurement in relation to people with learning disabilities has been conducted for research purposes, and has most frequently related to attempts to assess the relative effectiveness of services for people discharged from long-stay institutions. Exceptions to this would be work which has sought to evaluate special services, often for people with challenging behaviour (Murphy and Clare 1991; McGill *et al.* 1994) and a range of studies associated with the implementation of the All Wales Strategy (Welsh Office 1991; Evans *et al.* 1994; Allen and Lowe 1995). Many recent outcome measures are strongly influenced by the framework outlined by O'Brien and Lyle (1987), which is drawn from ideas about the right to lead an ordinary life and is based on the idea of five accomplishments:

- *Community presence* – to share with other citizens choices in respect of workplace, leisure, home and education.
- *Choice* – to make choices and benefit from experiences which guide choice among a variety of options in all areas of life.
- *Competence* – to develop competence which will increase independence and social skills.
- *Respect* – to gain respect from other members of the community by being supported in achieving valued social roles.
- *Community participation* – to form friendships and relationships with members of the local community.

Of course statements couched at this level of generality do not in themselves form an outcome measurement system but they can form useful signposts in deciding how to measure quality of life. Adaptations and additions have been suggested in the process of trying to develop workable systems for practice. For example, Evans and Gray (1990) modified this framework to produce a standards matrix with seven key elements involving, first, the addition of continuity and individuality and, second, an emphasis, within the domain of participation, on recognizing the differing depth and importance of some relationships. This matrix allowed each domain to be investigated along three dimensions: place of residence, daytime occupation and use of leisure time. Despite this level of detail, in a review of arrangements for routine evaluation, practitioners apparently reported that the standards matrix was found to be insufficiently operationalized to be of practical use (Henwood *et al.* 1993). The latter study also found that inspection units were often using instruments which had been developed largely for older people, which gives rise to considerable concern in the light of the numbers of group-specific instruments which could help to give an informed basis for inspection. With regard to routine practice, this inspection found no examples of the aggregation of review information from Individual Plans, although such reviews might initially be supposed to be a promising source of overall information about progress in services for people with learning disabilities.

Domains identified in research studies

Emerson and Hatton (1994) provide a comprehensive review of the literature in relation to research studies which have measured outcomes for service users. The review covers 70 publications (representing 45 studies) which have provided qualitative or quantitative data on user-related outcomes, most of which compare hospital-based institutional care and community-based staffed housing. Emerson and Hatton identify a number of general domains of outcome measurement and give examples of studies which have used each of them. Wright et al. (1994) identify similar broad domains which are:

- everyday functioning – adaptive and maladaptive behaviour;
- engagement or participation in meaningful activity;
- personal experience of life and life quality; and
- social relationships, networks and community participation.

These domain areas will be discussed in more depth.

Everyday functioning

This relates to the competence of service users and is most frequently measured using rating scales completed by staff, for example the Adaptive Behaviour Scale (Nihira et al. 1974). The ABS Part I, for example, asks staff to assess functioning in ten domains:

Independent functioning	Domestic activity
Physical development	Vocational activity
Economic activity	Self-direction
Language development	Responsibility
Numbers and time	Socialization

The Disability Assessment Schedule (DAS) (Holmes et al. 1982) covers similar areas and has been used in the UK for giving a descriptive profile of service populations but not (in its complete form) for outcome measurement as far as we are aware. Knapp et al. (1992) used part of the scale. Wright et al. (1994) report that one of the authors reviewed over 50 scales measuring everyday functioning and that the ABS scored best in relation to a set of criteria including coverage, comprehensiveness, validity, reliability, sensitivity and ease of use. There is general agreement that the evidence about adaptive behaviour shows that change in place of residence alone is insufficient to generate changes in skill levels.

There are various ways in which competence as reflected in these scales may be changed: changes in the environment, changes in the person's support system and changes in the person him or herself. Few scales explicitly allow in their scoring a distinction between functioning which is restricted by environmental factors and functioning which reflects the person's lack of capacity to undertake a task even in favourable environmental conditions. This harks back to a debate mentioned earlier: if we wish to use ABS scores to create matched groups of individuals with similar capabilities then we need a measure which ignores environmental considerations as far as possible. If, on the other hand, we wish to measure changes in functioning brought about by environmental change, then actual functioning in the given environment is what is needed (Wright et al. 1994).

In relation to challenging behaviour, or behaviour problems, while dramatic improvements may be achieved for some individuals, the evidence across the board is of no change, or even a worsening of such behaviour in the wake of deinstitutionalization (Knapp et al. 1992; Emerson and Hatton 1994). Both ABS and DAS contain sections measuring the existence and severity of behaviour problems. It is notoriously difficult to achieve satisfactory reliability across different raters in this area: Qureshi (1994) reviews some of the difficulties and solutions.

Engagement or participation in meaningful activity

This is normally measured by intensive observational studies which involve non-participant observers recording the type of activity in which people are engaged at regular time intervals throughout the day. In general, activity is classified under a number of headings, such as social interactions, appropriate or non-appropriate engagement, neutral activity and staff interactions (Felce 1986). The approach has been widely used (Mansell and Beasley 1990) although it is not without its critics, who have pointed to the lack of knowledge about what would constitute normal levels of engagement and the difficulties of avoiding effects on the behaviour of the people observed. These issues are discussed at length in Wright et al. (1994) where a more participative diary-based approach with a focus on one person for a whole day is recommended as an alternative.

In reviewing the range of studies that have used observational measures of engagement, Emerson and Hatton (1994) comment that they frequently lack adequate descriptive data concerning potentially significant facility and user characteristics: in short, they display the recurring problem of a failure to specify inputs in detail. Nonetheless, it seems that much variation in engagement levels can be accounted for by two factors: the competence of the service users and the amount of assistance (advice, prompting, guidance) received from staff. This is of significance because other evidence suggests that the degree to which staff intervene to give assistance has less to do with the numbers of staff or the staff/client ratios, than with the ethos and philosophy underlying care practices (Felce 1986). Proponents of an 'active support' model which entails clearly defined structures for planning staff and user activity have sometimes found that this has been perceived to be in conflict with ideas about user self-determination derived from a normalization perspective. They have argued that this is based on a misinterpretation, because social role valorization does involve assisting individuals to develop skills and appropriate behaviour as well as changing the service environment (Mansell *et al.* 1994; Emerson and Hatton 1994). It is generally assumed that engagement constitutes a desirable outcome for users, although there is little evidence about subjective evaluations by users of different degrees of engagement, partly at least because many of the clients studied had severe or profound learning disabilities.

Personal experience of life and life quality

A number of studies have addressed users' expressed satisfaction perhaps with services (Knapp *et al.* 1992) or quality of life more generally (Heal and Chadsey-Rusch 1985). The literature on regimes in residential care for older people illustrates the general point that features of a person's everyday life such as the choices available, should be assessed in relation to the specific individual, and not assumed to be a characteristic of the overall setting. Some people will exercise more choice than others in a given setting. O'Brien and Lyle argue that choice refers to the experience of autonomy both in relation to small everyday matters such as what to eat and what to wear, and to larger life-defining matters such as where to live and who to live with. All of these areas can be, and have been, translated into questions for outcome measurement (for example Schalock *et al.* 1989).

The issues around the collection of views directly from service users will be discussed in a later section. It is obviously of key importance to undertake this wherever possible. Quantitative structured scales for this purpose have tended to originate from the North American literature. The Lifestyle Satisfaction Scale (LSS) (Heal and Chadsey-Rusch 1985) contains four subscales reflecting:

Community satisfaction   Satisfaction with services
Friends and free-time satisfaction   General satisfaction

The report describes the scale as experimental but, within the confines of one study with volunteer subjects, demonstrated acceptable levels of test–retest and interrater reliability. This measure, which assesses subjective opinions of people with learning disabilities, may be contrasted with another quality of life scale, developed by Schalock *et al.* (1989), which uses mostly descriptive rather than evaluative items. Thus the LSS elicits examples of rules and asks whether people like them, while in contrast the Quality of Life Index asks people (among other things) how much control they have over various specified aspects of their life, but does not go on to ask their evaluation of this. Questions cover the areas of community involvement, social relations and environmental control. Both measures reflect a normative professional view of the domains of importance, but a decision to use one, or even both, would be dependent on the kind of information required, as well as the language skills and understanding of the proposed respondents.

Other instruments include the User Interview (Cambridge *et al.* 1991) which makes use of visual aids and which covers home environment, structured activities, social contacts and life satisfaction. An instrument designed for self-completion or completion by staff is the Life Experiences Checklist (Ager 1993) which is intended to be applicable to people whether or not they are disabled, and is a 50-item checklist which covers five domains:

Home	Freedom
Leisure	Opportunities
Relationships	

It has been used in studies of people with learning disabilities but it seems likely that it is generally completed by staff rather than the individuals concerned. Its use has reinforced other findings that people with learning disabilities have comparatively restricted social relationships and friendships, and that a move into ordinary housing in the community can, at least in the short term, worsen this by restricting the overall numbers of people immediately available to relate to on a day-to-day basis.

Social relationships, networks and community participation

Community participation and the support, or creation, of a range of social relationships seems to be one of the most difficult areas in which to achieve substantial progress. Participation in community-based activities is often measured by the inclusion of questions about the use of community-based facilities, such as banks, shops or pubs (de Kock *et al.* 1988). Other studies have looked more broadly at the degree of acceptance by the local community (McConkey *et al.* 1993), or at personal factors which might affect acceptance such as personal appearance and presentation (Knapp *et al.* 1992). The measurement of social relationships is a more difficult area. It is possible to use diary methods or interviews with staff to assess the number, type and frequency of social contacts. Flynn (1986) reports that in general people with learning disabilities could not reliably report the answers to factual questions about numbers and frequency, and might readily identify people as close friends, where their contact and relationship was extremely limited. They could of course discuss their satisfaction with existing relationships and say what they would like in future.

Emerson and Hatton (1994) identify a separate domain of outcomes which they characterize as general social indicators of quality of life. These include income (Walker *et al.* 1993), the physical environment (Felce *et al.* 1985) and number and type of personal possessions (Conneally *et al.* 1992). Emerson and Hatton conclude that these indicators are relatively underused, and that even where used they rarely embody a comparison with non-disabled people. Exceptions to this include Stanley and Roy (1988) who did make such a comparison, and found similar levels of life satisfaction and overall quality of life except in relation to the use of community facilities. Overall, Emerson and Hatton (1994: 11) argue that it is time to move away from standards of comparison which are related to the need to demonstrate the superiority of smaller community-based services over existing institutional provision, towards comparisons based on judgements about 'the adequacy, acceptability or decency of the quality of life experienced by people with learning disabilities'. Certainly work on the specification of outcomes which relate to the objectives of community-based services without an, at least implicit, comparison with institutional care, is relatively underdeveloped in the field, although some progress in outlining a conceptual model for a broader assessment of quality of life has been made by Felce and Perry (1995). These authors argue that personal satisfaction with life conditions is mediated through personal values and aspirations, to produce overall quality of life. They outline a model for the relationships between these aspects, and indicate the research and development agenda which would be required to see the approach carried through into practice. Felce and colleagues are currently considering a number of available measures, which purport to address similar dimensions of quality of life, and investigating whether or not the results agree if different measures are applied in the same situations.

Most studies of deinstitutionalization have used a range of measures, reflecting a belief that outcomes are multidimensional. None has attempted to construct a single quantitative indicator of quality of life. Knapp *et al.* (1992), for example, collected information on: skills; behaviour problems; satisfaction with social interactions; depression; morale. These areas were all measured using existing scales or parts of scales. Cheetham *et al.* (1992) comment that studies of community provision have commonly tended to assemble an eclectic selection of outcome measures, but warn that the advantages of using measures of proven reliability and validity may well be lost if, as in the PSSRU evaluation of *Care in the Community* demonstration projects, these scales are subsequently pruned and adapted in the course of building up the instrumentation for the particular study.

The influence of service users

With rare exceptions (such as Whittaker *et al.* 1991) service users have not been involved in determining the dimensions to be investigated in evaluations. Henwood *et al.* (1993) argued that the items of concern to users that were least likely to be addressed by existing instruments included:

- choice over where to live and who to live with;
- choice over staff and a say in new appointments;
- help in getting a job and proper wages for work;
- financial advice;
- opportunities for ordinary holidays;
- avoidance of professional jargon; and
- being treated as an equal by staff.

This document made a rare systematic attempt to compare the policy framework of the All Wales Strategy with instruments used for quality monitoring, and with a framework derived from literature on the views of service users. The report argued that an initial concern with quality of outcomes had to be broadened to include a focus on quality of process (that is, how users were treated by staff), because many of the concerns of users centred round these issues. This again reminds us that the distinction between process and outcome is not entirely clear-cut. In health literature, some authors seem understandably cynical about evaluations involving user views of process which thereby only concentrate on the 'hotel' aspects of the service (Pollitt 1987a; Donabedian 1992). However, it may be argued that, in community care, the way the service is delivered is an integral part of the service in an even stronger sense than it is in health care. In staffed housing, or a day centre, the way a person is treated on a daily basis is an integral part of their social environment for large parts of their life.

Eliciting the views of people with learning disabilities

A number of particular issues arise in relation to interviewing, or other-wise obtaining direct expressions of views from, people with learning disabilities (for a review see Prosser 1989; Booth *et al.* 1990). Many of these possible problems undoubtedly affect interviews in other contexts, that is they are not specific to people with learning disabilities, but they do feature with greater prominence in situations where people's understanding may be limited, or where socialization may have emphasized deference and discouraged criticism. The first obvious example is found where there are difficulties in discovering the views of people with limited or no language, or idiosyncratic forms of communication. This has led to the use of a range of techniques such as drawings of smiling and unsmiling faces to which people may point (Simons *et al.* 1989) or the use of photographs or other visual aids (Leedham 1989; Cambridge *et al.* 1991).

If people cannot be interviewed at all, then it may be necessary to rely on interviews with staff or carers, although this may be supplemented by observational techniques which can give an indication of some external features of quality of life, such as engagement in meaningful activity. Of course, observation can also supplement information collected directly from service users, but it has most frequently been used where the individuals involved have severe or profound learning disabilities and the main source of evidence would otherwise be staff report. In support of the need for such observational work, Felce (1986) cites evidence that staff may not be able to give an accurate account of the activity of residents even when they are filling in diaries to help in the process of collecting information.

Studies which rely on single structured interviews frequently find themselves conducting a large number of proxy interviews with carers. Todd *et al.* (1993) set out to collect consumers' views of the All Wales Strategy, but in the event, 92 per cent of interviews were conducted with parents or other relatives. Although it is certainly arguable that parents may be viewed as users of services, it is acknowledged that there may be differences of opinion between people with learning disabilities and their parents, and that there is a need where possible to collect the views of both parties separately (Grant 1992; Todd *et al.* 1992). In addition, there is some evidence that staff and parents may rate individuals differently: for example, Qureshi (1990) found that staff rated young adults' domestic skills more highly than did their parents. She speculated that this was because staff tended to rate according to the perceived capacity to undertake a task such as making a cup of tea, while parents made ratings according to whether the person actually did so in a normal domestic context. We do not have a research-based understanding of the degree to which the use of third-party informants produces information which is systematically different from that which might be obtained by direct elicitation, nor of differences between different people providing care.

Among people who can be interviewed there may be a failure to understand questions which are too abstract or too complicated. Whittaker *et al.* (1991: 72) indicated that the original question, 'Do the other people in the house understand about privacy?' was best changed to two specific questions: 'Do other people in the house knock before coming into your room?' and 'Is there a lock on the bathroom door?'. This study involved the evaluation of services by two people who were themselves learning disabled, with another person as a support, and provides a useful discussion of the practical problems to be overcome and the advantages of involving users as evaluators.

In trying to use structured questioning with closed options, problems may arise from question form and wording. Systematic research in the USA has demonstrated a tendency to acquiescence on the part of people with learning disabilities, which may reflect limited understanding or a desire to please the interviewer (Sigelman *et al.* 1981; Bercovici 1983). This does have the implication that answers to yes/no questions are likely to be biased and this has led some researchers to include specific subscales within life satisfaction instruments for detecting this bias (Heal and Chadsey-Rusch 1985). One way in which a tendency to deference may be countered more generally is the development of advocacy and self-advocacy schemes which are designed to assist people in being more assertive and in expressing their opinions (Simons 1993). In addition to acquiescence bias, there are also demonstrated effects of question form on responses, for example the tendency to choose the last of a range of multiple response choices (Sigelman *et al.* 1982).

Some commentators have favoured avoiding structured closed questioning altogether. However, other problems may arise in less structured interviewing, as a consequence of a tendency for people with learning disabilities to omit important features of context in discourse (Kernan and Sabsay 1984). This means that an interviewer who is a stranger may have difficulty in interpreting what is said. In general, guidelines for eliciting the views of people with learning disabilities recommend a period of observation and getting to know the person if possible, coupled with an interview which involves concrete questions with simple forms (Wyngaarden 1981; Flynn 1986). Obtaining informed consent is also raised as an issue which may need special attention. Although there are life-satisfaction and quality-of-life scales which have been developed for, and used with, this group of people, these are only likely to be suitable for use with those whose disability is not severe (Schalock *et al.* 1989; Heal and Chadsey-Rusch 1985). Communicating with people with severe or profound learning disabilities remains a difficulty to which there may be no generally applicable answers, but only a range of solutions suitable for particular individuals.

Difficulties in communication and possible solutions are summarized in Box 7.1.

Box 7.1   Potential difficulties in communication and possible solutions

Difficulties	Solutions
Limited or non-existent language skills	Non-verbal means of communication
Tendency towards acquiescence	Observation and getting to know the person
Influence of question format	Avoiding too structured an approach in interviewing
Omission of important contextual information	Advocates and self-advocacy
Deference	

Conclusions

This chapter has considered the domains currently in use in outcome measurement for people with learning disabilities. These demonstrate the continuing influence of ideas about the importance of an ordinary life, and in some ways are close to the spirit of the new legislation in the sense that emphasis is placed on individual opportunities for choice, developing competence and living in a homely domestic environment. Nonetheless, if the aim is to develop measures which will apply on a longer term and continuing basis, and to people living in the community, it may be time to develop beyond the implicit standard of comparison (institutional care) which leads to the translation of the concept of choice into questions about whether people can choose what to wear and what to eat, for example. Clearly these are basic conditions which must be satisfied, and perhaps should not be neglected in outcome measurement at present, but ideas about a normal life which involve comparison with people who are not disabled or institutionalized are gaining ground. Agreement about principles should not be overemphasized. Parents, for example, may value safety, and protection against abuse, more highly than independence and freedom of choice.

The difficulties which may arise in obtaining evaluative opinions from people with learning disabilities have to be recognized, and attempts made to overcome them where possible. Service users could be involved to a greater extent than they are at present. It would be valuable to develop further a knowledge base about likely biases if information is collected from third parties, and keep separate the collection of information about outcomes for carers and service users. The most appropriate method of collecting data needs to be carefully considered: it may be helpful to use observation or diary methods in preference to interviews where specific information is required, especially if numbers or frequencies are to be investigated. There is little evidence of the aggregation of individual information, say from individual plans, which might seem potentially usable. Reasons for reluctance to do this might fruitfully be investigated.

Summary

Ideas about the aspiration towards a normal life have probably had a stronger influence on practice with people who have learning disabilities than any other client group. The argument that the major long-term needs of individuals in this group are for social rather than medical care is well established. Most outcome measurement has been conducted in relation to the comparison of quality of life before and after discharge from long-stay hospital. Comparison with equivalent non-disabled groups living in the community is relatively neglected. Measurements by researchers regularly investigate skills, behaviour problems, the physical environment, meaningful occupation, expressed satisfaction, social activities and relationships. There is widespread acceptance of a set of common principles which emphasize the importance of community presence and participation, respect choice and competence, although parents, for example, may also wish to emphasize safety and protection from abuse. There is, however, still scope for disagreement about how these principles are translated into action, one instance being how to strike a balance between active intervention to teach individuals how to undertake valued social roles, and respecting the apparent choices of individuals who appear to wish not to do this. Routine data collection based on these principles does not seem to be widely occurring. Any scope for aggregating the structured collection of information about individuals, as in Individual Programme Plans (IPPs) and reviews, does not yet seem to have been realized.

There are difficulties in directly obtaining the views of people with learning disabilities. These reflect not only communication problems where people have no speech or language, but also, in many instances, an individual's past experiences in social or service environments which may not have encouraged assertiveness or a critical approach. There are difficulties in relying solely on the views of staff or family carers, although there is little systematic evidence about the kinds of bias which might be introduced by this. Recently, there are signs of much greater efforts to discover and take account of the views of service users and, more rarely, to involve them actively in the process of collecting information about outcomes. Users' views emphasize the importance of the process of service delivery, as mediated through staff attitudes and behaviour towards them, and the way in which this process shapes their social environment.

Further reading

Emerson, E. and Hatton, C. (1994) *Moving Out: relocation from hospital to community*. London: HMSO.
  Comprehensive review of research studies of relocation (all studies published between 1980 and 1993). Gives detail of outcome measures used and common findings.
Felce, D. and Perry, J. (1995) Quality of life: its definition and measurement. *Research in Developmental Disabilities*, 16(4): 51–74.
  Outlines a framework for looking at quality of life for people with learning disability which draws on the general literature on quality of life.
Wright, K., Leedham, I. and Haycox, A. (1994) *Evaluating Community Care: services for people with learning difficulties*. Buckingham: Open University Press.
  Describes the principles involved in evaluating community care services. Various chapters consider the definition and measurement of outcomes, and the measurement of costs.

CHAPTER 8

CARERS

Introduction

The work of informal carers, and the difficulties they face, have been increasingly recognized in recent years. *Caring for People* noted that practical support for carers should be a high priority in the new community care arrangements and that services should respond flexibly and sensitively to carers' needs. The subsequent Carers (Recognition and Services) Act 1995 introduced the obligation for local authorities to carry out an assessment of carers' own needs, when requested by carers to do so. In the light of these policy developments, it is necessary that any evaluation of community care outcomes should take full account of the impact of community care for carers.

Needs and objectives

As outlined in Chapter 3, carers have identified a variety of different services that they need: information and advice, practical help, opportunities for time off, financial assistance, emotional support and a choice about whether to continue caring (Carers' Alliance, n.d.; King's Fund 1988; Richardson *et al.* 1989; London Research Centre 1991; NCVO 1992). Underpinning these identified needs is the sense that carers should receive proper recognition of their work, experience, knowledge and individual needs. The lack of particular services will affect different carers in different ways, and outcome measures need to take account of the full range of their needs.

It has to be recognized that tensions will sometimes arise between different policy objectives, and that carers' needs may conflict with those of the people for whom they are providing care (Perring et al. 1990). A wish to avoid the use of institutional care, for instance, may result in unacceptable burdens for carers, and enabling carers to cease caring should itself be a valid goal (Twigg et al. 1990). On the other hand, a wish to facilitate independent living may conflict with carers' wishes to continue providing care, or cut across carers' concerns about safety and protection for people who are vulnerable. Such issues need to be addressed at both policy and practice level, and are relevant to decisions about which outcomes are to be measured.

Consideration of community care outcomes should not focus solely on negative aspects: caring can also have a positive side (Perring et al. 1990; Grant and Nolan 1993), which could be either enhanced or weakened by the provision or lack of appropriate community care services. In relation to parents caring for disabled children, for example, the emphasis in the literature has changed from a focus on the supposed pathological effects on the family of the presence of a child with learning disability, towards a more positive emphasis on the ways in which parents cope and their evaluations of the reliability, sufficiency and suitability of services (Byrne and Cunningham 1985; Sloper et al. 1991; Qureshi 1992; Beresford 1994).

Measuring outcomes

Caring can have an impact on many aspects of carers' lives. Toseland et al. (1990) cite a number of effects on psychological, social and physical well-being. Psychological difficulties include depression, anxiety, anger, frustration, excessive guilt, a sense of lack of competence, and self-blame. Carers may feel lonely and isolated and lack social support. Caring can lead to conflicts within families about caring responsibilities and can adversely affect relationships between carers and the people for whom they are providing care. Sleep disturbance, lack of appetite, psychosomatic complaints and physical ill-health can occur. Not least, caring can have important practical effects in relation to the loss of employment, loss of earnings and additional expenditure (Parker 1990). Such losses may or may not be willingly accepted, but there is a sense in which they may be considered to be outcomes of caring.

It has been assumed that these various impacts of caring can influence carers' willingness or ability to continue to provide care, although as will be outlined there is a complex set of relationships between these impacts, the perceived strain of caring, carers' psychological health and a decision to accept alternatives to family care. There has been considerable debate about the degree to which costs and benefits to carers are or should be incorporated into studies of the cost-effectiveness of services (Ungerson 1995), and a number of research studies have attempted to develop ways to cost carers' contributions (Wright 1987; Netten 1989). Evaluative research studies which have included outcome measurement for carers have been primarily interested in the effects of services on carers' levels of stress (interpreted, as will be outlined, in a variety of ways) and on their willingness to continue caring.

Box 8.1   Approaches to measuring outcomes for carers

- Semi-structured (with ratings carried out by interviewer): for example, in the areas of subjective burden, extent of strain, mental health difficulties, social life, household routine, employment, financial affairs, child-related difficulties, physical health difficulties (Challis and Davies 1986)
- Standard measures: for example, focusing on distress, burden, strain, stress or malaise

---

In research on carers, two different approaches to assessing impacts have been adopted (Box 8.1). The first, particularly common in studies in the 1960s and 1970s, was to use a semi-structured approach to examine a number of domains or specific tasks, with the interviewer then rating whether a burden or problem existed (Grad and Sainsbury 1968; Hoenig and Hamilton 1969; Stevens 1972). This approach was subsequently developed to distinguish between practical tasks or presenting difficulties on the one hand, and the extent to which these were perceived as burdens by carers themselves (Creer et al. 1982). A semi-structured approach does have the advantage of being able to explore broad areas in as much detail as is appropriate to individual situations. Grad and Sainsbury (1968) argued that validity was obtained through the selection of items that could be objectively defined, and that their pilot study achieved high inter-rater reliability. More recently, MacCarthy et al. (1989) found that interviewer ratings correlated well with the total scores obtained using the General Health Questionnaire (described below) and Present State Examination (see Chapter 6).

The studies by Grad and Sainsbury (1968) and Hoenig and Hamilton (1969) provided the basis for Challis and Davies' (1986) evaluation of outcomes for informal carers in the Kent Community Care Scheme. Using three-point scales to reflect the extent of difficulty experienced, they examined a total of nine items:

Subjective burden	Employment
Extent of strain	Financial affairs
Mental health difficulties	Child-related difficulties
Social life	Physical health difficulties
Household routine	

The data enabled the researchers to establish statistically significant differences in outcome for carers in the community care scheme on the first three items, as compared with a control group.

The second approach involves the use or development of standard measures to examine specific aspects of the caring task. Some studies have used a battery of measures to explore a number of domains in detail. Others have developed short scales which incorporate several different domains. In many cases, studies have focused on just one or two issues such as distress, burden, strain, stress or malaise.

It is important, though, to be clear exactly what is meant by such terms, what is being measured, and how it relates to the caring task as a whole. Nolan and Grant (1992) point out, for example, that 'burden' and 'stress' are vague concepts – even though others have sought to define 'burden' as 'the presence of problems, difficulties or adverse events which affect the lives of significant others' (Platt 1985) or 'that element of family hardship that is explicitly attributed to the patient' (Gibbons *et al.* 1984). Certainly it is important to distinguish between measures which seek to reflect the perceived impact of caring (which usually list tasks or problems and ask for carers' responses to these), as opposed to global measures of psychological distress (usually measured through checklists of psychosomatic symptoms).

Box 8.2   Objective and subjective dimensions of caring

- Objective: practical tasks, aspects of behaviour, changes in family relations, employment or health
- Subjective: emotional reactions, perceptions of strain, reduced morale, anxiety and depression

---

With regard to the impact of caring, Grad and Sainsbury (1963) proposed a distinction between 'objective' and 'subjective' burden (Box 8.2), and argued that there was an often implicit assumption of a causal relationship between the two. Within this distinction, objective burden refers to practical or concrete events such as changes in the behaviour of the persons for whom care is provided, resultant practical problems and tasks for carers, as well as changes in family relations, employment and health (Morris *et al.* 1988b). Subjective burden then refers to carers' emotional reactions, perceptions of strain, reduced morale, anxiety and depression related to caring. However, the relationship between the two is far from clear: objective factors may be distressing but not burdensome, or they may be differentially burdensome for different people (Platt 1985; Nolan and Grant 1992). Equally, levels of psychological distress, as reflected in symptom checklists, may not be a consequence of caring at all, but may be related to other factors in people's lives.

It is established in the carer literature that the relationship between objective measures, such as the level of impairment of the cared-for person or the kind and frequency of tasks performed, is less closely related to carers' perceptions of burden than might have been supposed. One prominent response to this has been the development of work on styles of coping, where stress is conceptualized as a process through which the individual assesses potential stressors and brings to bear a variety of resources to deal with them (see, for example, Quine and Pahl 1989; Sloper et al. 1991; Beresford 1994). Thus individual styles of coping are seen as mediating between external factors and a person's responses. This more positive model, of people actively constructing their own ways of living and dealing with difficulties, has been less frequently applied to people in receipt of services than to carers.

Although carers do cope differentially with apparently similar circumstances, nonetheless there are some consistent findings in the carer literature about the relationship between particular features of the caring situation and outcomes. These findings are valuable in indicating important dimensions for assessment of carers' needs as well as areas for outcome measurement. For example, the presence of severe behaviour problems on the part of the cared-for person has been widely demonstrated to influence both carers' levels of distress and the eventual decision to seek alternatives to family care (Gilleard et al. 1984; Levin et al. 1989; Quine and Pahl 1989). In general, behaviour problems are more important in this respect than, for example, levels of physical impairment of the cared-for person. There is an increasing recognition that practical tasks in themselves, may be a relatively unimportant factor in the creation of distress (Nolan and Grant 1992), except when their performance imposes high opportunity costs or, for example, involves loss of sleep. Rather, it may be more subtle, personal and less easily measurable concerns, such as the loss of a personal relationship or anxiety about a person's future, that underpin the problem and therefore need to be explored and dealt with if distress is to be reduced (Perring et al. 1990).

It is important to recognize that the link between carer distress and the wish to seek alternative sources of care is not straightforward. Parents of adults with learning disability may seek alternatives to family care because they believe this is consistent with ideas about independence and a normal life, and not as a consequence of their own distress. Qureshi (1993) identified carers' opportunity costs, particularly in relation to foregone employment, as an important factor related to the wish to find alternatives to family care, while distress, as measured by the Malaise Inventory, was not related to the wish for alternative care. In addition, it is helpful to note that relatives' expressed willingness to accept residential care is a far better predictor of eventual placement in such care than many other factors, including levels of distress (Levin et al. 1989; Askham and Thompson 1990).

This suggests that a single-minded focus on outcomes such as reducing psychological distress in carers will not necessarily achieve a hoped-for reduction in the numbers seeking residential alternatives.

It is evident, therefore, that it is important to understand the interrelationships between different dimensions and not simply to treat all outcomes as separate factors. Nolan *et al.* (1990) suggest an extended model involving environment, stress and malaise: this provides a means for exploring direct relationships between different factors within each of the three categories. Nolan and Grant (1992) argue that the 'final outcomes' of caring should be measured in terms of emotional or physical health (or malaise): other impacts, such as a poor social life or change in relationships, would then represent intermediate stages along this path, but with no certainty that malaise would result. The understanding of structural relationships between outcomes would seem to represent an advance on situations where emotional distress or physical ill-health are simply seen as further aspects of the impact of caring – alongside other dimensions such as practical tasks, coping with difficult behaviour, disruption to family life, impact on social and personal life, employment and finances. However, understanding of these other dimensions, and their relationship to service inputs, is required before outcome measurement can be used to decide on appropriate interventions.

Specific measures

A large number of measures have been used to assess the impact of caring on informal carers either on a single occasion or over a period of time. Some studies have examined outcomes in relation to the provision of a specific service, such as respite care or domiciliary support, and some have involved control groups. The measures have most frequently focused on emotional health, depression or morale, and three of the more common measures will be discussed below. Studies that use a package of measures themselves tend to explore a number of psychological variables in detail. Lawton *et al.* (1989), for instance, measured depression, positive and negative affect, subjective burden, positive gains from caring and own perceptions of competence; Toseland *et al.* (1990) examined not only affect and burden but also psychiatric symptoms, informal and formal social supports, and the relationship between carers and the people for whom they were providing care; while Fadden *et al.* (1987) assessed role function, distress, disturbed behaviour, level of coping and degree of perceived control. Not surprisingly, the use of a large number of measures can mean that their completion can take up to 2 hours.

Other studies have developed their own measures. Zarit *et al.* (1980) used a 29-item self-report inventory which looked at the carer's health, psychological well-being, finances, social life and relationship with the person for whom care was being provided. As Nolan and Grant (1992) point out, however, the value of the summed scores derived from the inventory is questionable, given that it contains a variety of disparate items as well as implicit assumptions that particular impacts on carers' lives automatically represent sources of stress. Nolan and Grant themselves developed a self-completion Carers' Assessment of Difficulties Index (CADI). This contains 30 items of difficulty that carers may experience, but includes an assessment of whether these items are in fact stressful for the carers themselves, thus attempting to separate subjective and objective aspects. Morris *et al.* (1988a) designed both an intimacy questionnaire and a strain scale.

A different approach was adopted by Mohide *et al.* (1988), who examined the social, physical and emotional burdens of caring in relation to the broad amounts of time that carers experienced such burdens. The specific factors examined included the relationship with the person for whom care was being provided, socialization, physical well-being, sleep, and freedom from anxiety and frustration. A time trade-off technique was then used to determine the extent to which respondents would trade off length of life (in their present circumstances) against improved quality of life (but for a shorter time-span). The approach enabled numeric utility scores to be calculated to indicate the degree of carer burden and overall quality of life. The instrument itself was administered by trained interviewers and took an average of 20 minutes to complete.

As has been indicated above, though, many studies have used one or two existing measures, either with or without original instruments of their own. Box 8.3 gives an indication of the measures used in a small sample of studies.

It has to be noted that the use of particular measures does not in itself give any indication of their usefulness or appropriateness for measuring outcomes. Some, for instance, will have been designed for specific circumstances, as in the case of the Relatives' Stress Scale (RSS), which was intended for use with carers of people with dementia (Greene *et al.* 1982). While the studies cited in Box 8.3 give fuller details about the origins, content and applicability of the measures used, three of those measures will be briefly reviewed here.

The General Health Questionnaire (GHQ)

The GHQ is by far the most commonly used measure in the studies that have been reviewed. The GHQ (Goldberg 1972) is designed to identify four principal elements of distress:

Anxiety   Social dysfunction
Depression   Somatic symptoms related to malaise

Box 8.3   A selection of studies using a small number of measures to assess impacts or outcomes for carers

Category of persons receiving care	Authors	Measures used
Older people	Davies et al. 1990	Malaise Inventory
	Nolan and Grant 1992	Malaise Inventory Carers' Assessment of Difficulties Index
Older people with mental health problems	Eagles et al. 1987	60-item General Health Questionnaire Relatives' Stress Scale Relatives' Mood Scale
	Gilhooly 1984	Kutner Morale Scale OARS mental health scale
	Gilleard et al. 1984	30-item General Health Questionnaire Problem checklist
	Gilleard 1987	30-item General Health Questionnaire* Strain scale*
	Levin et al. 1989	28-item General Health Questionnaire* Social Behaviour Assessment Schedule*
	Morris et al. 1988	Strain scale Beck Depression Inventory Intimacy questionnaire
	Wattis et al. 1994	Relatives' Stress Scale*
People with mental health problems	Gibbons et al. 1984	28-item General Health Questionnaire Social Behaviour Assessment Schedule
	McCreadie et al. 1987	28-item General Health Questionnaire Social Adjustment Scale Self-Report
	Shanks and Gillen 1992	28-item General Health Questionnaire*
People with acute stroke	Greveson and James 1991	Caregiver Strain Index
Disabled children	Bradshaw and Lawton 1978	Malaise Inventory
	Quine and Pahl 1985	Malaise Inventory
	Romans-Clarkson et al. 1986	60-item General Health Questionnaire Interview Schedule for Social Interaction

* Measure was used on more than one occasion with the same respondents

The shorter versions comprise selected questions from the original 60-item schedule. One notable difference between GHQ-30 and GHQ-28 is that the latter includes four questions about suicidal thoughts whereas the former only includes one: this is an important consideration where such thoughts are not a primary concern of the study and where several such questions might only produce discomfort for the respondent. A 12-item version is also available. Keady and Nolan (1994) recommend the use of the GHQ as an adjunct to their proposed carer-led assessment system (CLASP), although they do not state a preferred version.

Levin et al. (1989) found that GHQ scores decreased for carers where the person they had been caring for had either died or been admitted to institutional care, whereas there was a slight increase for those who continued to provide care. Gilleard (1987) similarly noted a decreased score where the person being cared for was receiving day hospital care (or had been admitted to long-term institutional care). Eagles et al. (1987) found that, while carers of older people with dementia did not have significantly different GHQ scores from carers of people without dementia, RSS scores were significantly higher for the first group. This study emphasizes that the GHQ is not a measure of the stress of caring as such, and that there is no one-to-one relationship between global measures of distress, as reflected in symptom checklists, and measures of the strain of providing care, as perceived by carers.

The Social Behaviour Assessment Schedule (SBAS)

Like the GHQ, the SBAS (Platt et al. 1980) measures emotional distress. Unlike the GHQ, though, it also assesses disturbed behaviour and altered social performance on the part of the person for whom care is being provided, together with the impact of the social context and major life events on carers and other household members. The SBAS aims to establish correlations between these aspects.

The schedule takes the form of a 52-item standardized semi-structured interview. For each item, the interviewer rates the severity of the 'objective' difficulty and uses a four-point distress scale to measure the informant's emotional reaction. The distress scores have been found to be highly correlated with GHQ scores (Gibbons et al. 1984; Levin et al. 1989), and the authors of the schedule have tested its psychometric properties (Platt et al. 1980). Although the schedule is designed for use with the carers of people with mental health problems, the authors state that, with some small amendments and additions, it could be adapted to examine the impact of physical illness or other chronic conditions. It would also be possible to obtain details of the 'objective' problems direct from the disabled person rather than from a carer.

The Malaise Inventory (MI)

The Malaise Inventory, for its part, does not seek to differentiate between the impact of the circumstances or characteristics of the people for whom care is being provided, those of carers themselves, or the influence of external factors (Davies *et al.* 1990). Like the GHQ, it is essentially a checklist of symptoms, designed as a screening instrument for the study of psychiatric morbidity. The schedule, which was developed by Rutter *et al.* (1970), consists of 24 yes/no questions about emotional or physical states with an important psychological component. The total number of affirmative answers represents the overall malaise score. While the four studies cited in Box 8.3 used the MI to measure stress, none of them used it on more than one occasion with the same respondents in order to examine its sensitivity to change.

Some doubts have been raised about the precise meaning of the overall malaise scores. Hirst (1983) calculated that there was no single dimension, such as emotional disturbance, which underpinned those scores: it would therefore not be possible to locate different scores on a single meaningful scale. While Bebbington and Quine (1987) subsequently suggested that the final scores do reflect a unidimensional scale of stress, Nolan and Grant (1992) preferred a split into two sub-scales representing psychological and physical malaise, although this did not apply to all groups of carers. This does not alter the fact that different items and different scales may be measuring different aspects of stress, as found by Hirst and Bradshaw (1983).

Conclusions

Much work on outcomes for carers has measured distress, perceived strain of caring and the ending of informal care. This has reflected policy and practice objectives concerned largely with maintaining informal care, with an underlying, but questionable, assumption that the ending of informal care was often a consequence of the 'breakdown' of caring relationships in the face of intolerable pressures. Carers' organizations have criticized the targeting of help only on situations in danger of breakdown as 'rewarding failure to manage' and argued that carers should have a right to expect support even if they are determined to continue to provide care themselves. It would seem reasonable to argue that the achievement of a normal life, choice and independence are desirable objectives for carers as well as service users. To reinforce this argument, the research described in this chapter indicates that attention to carers' capacity to live a normal life, for example to take employment if they so choose, or to enjoy a social life, will be likely to enhance willingness to continue to provide care. Any practical approach to looking at outcomes for carers should include some attention to the positive satisfactions of caring, and how to work to increase them.

In addition, the monitoring of levels of distress or perceived strain may indicate the need for appropriate practical and emotional support to be directed at, for example, ensuring carers have enough sleep, or are assisted in coping with behaviour problems. If outcomes are measured then the relative success of interventions designed to achieve reduced levels of stress can be determined. In addition, the effects on carers of changes in service provision for service users will be evident from outcome monitoring. Clearly there is room for more work on understanding the impacts on carers of various forms of service provision, whether these services are provided directly for carers or for service users.

In discussing assessment for carers, Nolan and Grant (1992) and Grant and Nolan (1993) emphasize that it is essential to obtain carers' own views about the problems they face and not to assume, for instance, that the level of a person's physical dependency is a valid proxy for the amount of stress experienced by carers. We would certainly endorse this view. Service provision that is based on such limited dependency criteria could result in service needs not being fully recognized, with the danger that carers' stress levels or wish for alternative care could even increase as a result.

As was noted earlier, caring can involve difficult physical tasks, adversely affect family relationships, restrict social and personal life, disrupt employment and impose financial difficulties (Perring *et al.* 1990). However, distress and the wish for alternatives to family care may be related to qualitatively different features of the caring situation and to different service inputs. This illustrates the importance of understanding the relationships between inputs and outcomes, and the structural relationships between outcomes, before making recommendations about appropriate services. There is no reason to expect these relationships to be the same across all groups of carers. The relationship to the person cared for, the reason for care and the stage in the carer's life cycle will no doubt underlie important variations.

Summary

Informal caring can affect many aspects of carers' lives: employment opportunities, earnings, expenditure, sleep, appetite, physical ill-health and psychological well-being. It can also have positive effects, for instance in terms of the relationship between the carer and the person for whom care is being provided.

Some studies have adopted a qualitative, open-ended approach to assess carers' needs. Others have used a semi-structured format, with interviewers then rating responses on predetermined scales. A third approach has been to use either a range of standard measures or single instruments to examine specific impacts of the caring role. The emphasis in the latter case has most commonly been on aspects such as distress, stress or malaise. An important distinction to be made in measurement is between global measures of psychological distress based on symptom checklists and specific measures of the perceived strain of caring. The links between stress and a willingness to continue caring are by no means clear. Focusing just on aspects such as stress or strain also fails to address the other outcomes of caring, some of which may be positive. The multifaceted nature of the caring task must be reflected in any outcome evaluation if the full impact of caring is to be adequately addressed.

Further reading

Moriarty, J. and Levin, E. (1993) Interventions to assist caregivers. *Reviews in Clinical Gerontology*, 3: 301–308.
    This review considers the evidence for the effectiveness of a range of social care services designed to assist carers of older people.
Nolan, M., Grant, G. and Keady, J. (1996) *Understanding Family Care*. Buckingham: Open University Press.
    Draws together the results of the authors' substantial research on caring, with an emphasis on understanding the dynamics of caring relationships, and the satisfactions as well as the difficulties involved.
Qureshi, H. (1993) Impact on families, in C. Kiernan (ed.) *Research to Practice: learning disabilities and challenging behaviour*, pp. 89–118. Kidderminster: British Institute of Learning Disability.
    This paper discusses the factors influencing psychological distress and the desire for alternatives to family care in a sample of parents caring for adult children who had severe learning disabilities and challenging behaviour.

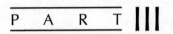

PART III

CONCLUSION

CHAPTER 9

TOWARDS OUTCOMES IN PRACTICE

Introduction

Two fundamental themes emerge from our reading of the literature and consideration of what is meant by community care (Box 9.1). The first concerns the shift towards the greater centrality of users and carers in the evaluation of community care outcomes. The second emphasizes the specific objectives of community care that need to be reflected in outcome measurement and to be distinguished from the focus of many existing measures. After discussing these two issues, this final chapter will consider some of the problems that may be encountered in the routine application of outcome measurement. For example, what are the incentives and obstacles to the collection and use of outcome information by professionals in their day-to-day practice? We will conclude by provisionally identifying some areas that require further research or development work if the measurement of community care outcomes is to become a reality.

Box 9.1   Principles underpinning the measurement of community care outcomes

- Users and carers should have a major role in judging the success of community care
- Need to take account of the objectives of community care: a normal life, choice, independence, having a say

---

User and carer involvement

One of the aims of *Caring for People* is to give service users a greater say in how they lead their lives. Services, for their part, must respond flexibly to the needs of both users and carers. The Health Committee argued that outcome measurement should follow the same principle and be undertaken 'from the perspective of those who use the service and their carers': they should have 'the major role' in identifying the relevant criteria for judging the success of the new community care policy (House of Commons 1993: paras 1, 7). This view echoes the calls for consumers to be seen as citizens (Pollitt 1988), for users' unique perspectives on services to be used to improve quality (Donabedian 1992), for user participation in service monitoring (Centre for Policy on Ageing 1990), and for researchers and users to work together (Oliver 1987; Barnes 1992).

The new arrangements thus indicate a clear shift in balance, away from the dominance of professionals and towards the views of users and carers. Nevertheless, we recognize that this is by no means unproblematic. Public expectations include the control of socially undesirable behaviour, thereby in some cases overruling the wishes of individual service users. Publicly-funded admissions to residential care are to depend on professional assessments of need, rather than users' wishes. Policy objectives (such as encouraging independence) may themselves conflict with the wishes of service users (who may, for instance, prefer tasks to be carried out by others). It is important not to generate naive expectations of homogeneity among users, but to recognize diversity and difference. Service users and carers from the various minority ethnic groups, for instance, will have ideas about what constitutes a normal life, or a desirable level of independence, which may or may not differ from prevailing views in the wider society. Moreover, user participation in general is not an end in itself, nor can it be achieved without effort. Some service users are vulnerable and in need of protection. Others may be especially deferential towards service providers, and it may be unreasonable to expect them to participate fully in planning or evaluation without the collective support of other users and support in acquiring the skills of self advocacy. Work by Goss and Miller (1995) suggests that in some authorities there is a genuine commitment towards a shift of power towards users and carers, and a recognition of the need to tackle the difficulties this can bring. In others, this is less evident.

The distribution of power among stakeholders will ultimately be an important influence on decisions about outcome monitoring. Services, for example, have to be targeted on those in greatest need, but this carries the corollary that 'lesser' needs may not be met. Given finite resource levels, who is to determine which needs are to be met and which objectives are the most important? The high satisfaction levels often reported for users and carers might be substantially reduced if more information were available about the possibilities that exist to provide additional or better services: how does a Social Services Department (SSD) balance the ethical need to share information and facilitate the participation of users and carers against the increased demands that may then result? Nor does the range of stakeholders comprise just users, carers and professional and managerial staff. Other potentially interested parties include those whose needs have not been identified and those for whom existing services are inappropriate or unacceptable – not to mention the general public which ultimately provides the resources. The interests of these many groups have to be recognized.

These problems underpin the process of outcome measurement and a value-free approach is not possible. Indeed, it may be that, in some cases, consensus may be unattainable and people will have to agree to differ. Nevertheless, the new arrangements do make it plain that the clarification of objectives is not to be simply a matter for SSD managers: users and carers, in particular, need to be centrally involved. This applies at all stages of the process: in identifying the issues to be examined, establishing the relative importance of different aspects, determining how to measure them, and (as is beginning to happen in some authorities) involving users in service evaluation.

In this book, we have reviewed some of the available literature on users' and carers' views about community care, which we have placed alongside the work that has already been carried out on outcome measurement. In many instances the measures reviewed may be useful in themselves or, as is more likely, their content could be helpful in indicating precisely which dimensions might be worth exploring, and what might constitute evidence of the impact of services. A good deal of further work will be required if outcome measures are to fully reflect users' and carers' views. Developing appropriate measures will involve the need to recognize and address possible conflicts between users, carers and a variety of professional staff. Henwood et al.'s (1993) approach (of listing and comparing the aspects considered important by different stakeholders) offers one way of becoming aware of the differences between interest groups. While this approach could no doubt be more widely applied, additional development work would still be required to resolve those differences and develop practical measures in particular local contexts. The example already cited in Trafford (1993) does show that a set of outcome criteria can be jointly agreed, even if that particular example relates just to residential care for older people. It remains to be demonstrated how staff and users might jointly develop monitoring systems to record inputs and outcomes for community care more generally. Such a development nonetheless seems essential if systems are to be properly focused, relevant to policy objectives for users and carers, and actually implemented.

The scope of outcome measurement in community care

It is clear from our review that community care covers a wide range of aspects of people's lives: to say it is multifaceted is surely an understatement. As we have seen, users and carers often want the term to include not just the care purchased or provided by SSDs but also services relating to housing, health and transport. Department of Health guidance stresses the need for effective collaboration, recognizing that many agencies have an impact on the quality of community care provided for users. The boundary between health and social services is a particularly grey area, and one that may be indistinguishable (and possibly unimportant) to many users: there is therefore an argument for examining outcomes for people who receive complex packages of care across community health and social care as a whole. It may well be that some impacts are achieved only by services acting in combination (Levin *et al.* 1989).

In community care, unlike acute health care, it cannot be assumed that the intended outcome of a specific service is identical for all who receive it. Respite or short-term care, for example, may be intended either to enhance the willingness of carers to continue providing care at home or to provide a bridge to long-term residential care and thereby enable the carer to gradually 'let go'. A single service could also have a range of different outcomes or impacts (both intended and unintended) in different areas of people's lives. To concentrate on specific aspects runs the risk of ignoring the possibility of (potentially more important) outcomes in other areas (Fitzpatrick 1992a). Yet to seek to encompass all the potential areas of impact may raise other problems. In the first place, it may be experienced as intrusive: what right does an agency have to expect users and carers to provide detailed information about their lives? Secondly, the length of the necessary measures would be daunting – and effectively impractical in agencies whose resources are already stretched to provide direct services: the opportunity costs of such an approach would be considerable. Clearly there is a balance to be struck which must involve ways of deciding with users and carers on the most important dimensions to measure in particular cases, while keeping within some broadly consistent overall structure which reflects the shortfalls that SSDs are willing or able to meet.

The evaluation of long-term and continuing care differs from the evaluation of short-term health care interventions, such as surgery or drug treatment. Although long-term care may sometimes involve interventions directed at the achievement of specific outcomes, aspects of process often represent important and continuing influences on user and carer satisfaction and quality of life. Harding and Beresford (1995) consulted a wide range of user organizations about what they wanted from social services staff. In addition to attaching importance to quality of service and skills of staff, respondents particularly emphasized the quality of relationships with staff. Although we argue for a shift towards a greater focus on outcomes, we would not wish to deny the importance of efforts to improve process. However, although some aspects of process may be important in themselves, others are implicitly justified by a belief that they lead to superior final outcomes. In an area such as social care, where process–outcome relationships are so uncertain, a focus on monitoring service process alone is not sufficient.

In the health sector, the incorporation of outcome data collection into routine practice has proved problematic but not impossible, at least in one particular experiment in a hospital setting (Bardsley and Coles 1992). In community care services, however, there are considerable difficulties in the way of meeting the conditions which facilitated success in the study described by Bardsley and Coles. Those conditions were: a focus on single conditions susceptible to intervention; professional consensus about likely recovery periods and possible complications; and a pre-existing general health status measure derived from work with patients. This book has demonstrated that these conditions are unlikely to be met in much of social care.

Developing outcome measures for community care

The usefulness of existing measures and approaches

We have argued that there is no off-the-shelf solution to the question of outcome measurement in community care, and that there is a need for continuing research and development work to address the issue of how to measure the central objectives of community care for individuals: a normal life, choice, independence, and having a say. An encouraging sign is that it is possible to identify an increasing number of research and development initiatives which are beginning to address these issues in a practical context. In addition, there is a knowledge base about outcome measurement, and also evidence about the diffusion and utilization of such knowledge, which potentially has much to contribute to efforts to establish the monitoring of effectiveness on a routine basis.

Part II of this book reviewed a number of measures and approaches that might potentially inform the measurement of community care outcomes. A common feature of many of those measures is that they have been developed in health care settings (Box 9.2). There may well be a degree of overlap between the issues they examine and the issues that are of concern in community care. Nevertheless, the extent of overlap is often limited and the underlying focus of concern generally different. Such considerations indicate a need for caution when considering the use of measures in a setting and for a purpose other than those for which they were designed.

As mentioned in Chapter 5, reviews of assessment instruments to decide whether they may be suitable for outcome measurement are a potentially valuable way forward (Ramsay *et al.* 1995).

Box 9.2   The measures currently available

Limitations
Focus is mainly on health care, not community care
Often designed for one-off assessments rather than measuring outcomes
Process of development seldom involved users and carers

Possible contributions
Some measures may be relevant to community care: for instance, in relation to morale, quality of life, stress, distress, and the ability to carry out activities of daily living
Work in progress seeks to measure social life and integration

---

Provided that existing measures address issues identified by users and carers as relevant to the new community care arrangements, there is no reason why they should not be used, in whole or in part, to inform the measurement of community care outcomes. Morale, general health, quality of life, stress, distress, or the ability to carry out activities of daily living may need to be examined: further work could build on the measures already available. Work is also taking place on the measurement of social life and integration, though adequate measures have yet to be produced. Despite the lack of ready-made outcome measures, much of the material we have included in this review – together with the results of other evaluations of specific types of services – might usefully inform the development of outcome measures by SSDs themselves.

Chapter 2 indicated that managers tend to prefer quantitative information because it can be aggregated and is sometimes thought to reflect a more scientific approach to measurement. It also links more easily into the requirements of financial systems. Front-line professionals, however, tend to prefer more qualitative open-ended measurement which leaves room for professional judgements and for the infinite variety of individual human needs. One important task is to investigate whether there are fruitful ways of combining these approaches. Two possibilities suggest themselves. One is to design review instruments which are largely open-ended but which contain a few closed sections that will provide the structured information necessary for management: a process of experiment and evaluation is called for to determine the optimum level of structure and the type of aggregated information that is really needed and that could be used for management and planning. Secondly, it may be possible to collect a few fairly crude quantitative indicators, while accepting that their interpretation may be problematic. Their purpose would simply be to raise questions to explore in subsequent in-depth studies: these could then seek to explain in detail any apparent differences between teams or areas in outcomes or activities by asking open-ended questions of those involved. Such qualitative approaches also have a role in exploratory work – for example, in finding out how people make judgements about the value of services to them, or for detecting unanticipated outcomes which have not been built into quantitative measures. Furthermore, qualitative approaches offer a means to gather contextual data which may provide invaluable information about the links between outcomes and inputs. Of course, knowledge about such links cannot be used to improve practice unless clear and consistent definitions of inputs, such as care management, are being used.

Addressing the objectives of the new community care arrangements

We have noted that issues of empowerment, independence, choice and personal control underpin the new community care arrangements. Such considerations are rarely addressed within measures of health care outcomes and they represent largely uncharted territory. One partial exception is the 'Five Accomplishments' approach, used in the field of learning disability (O'Brien and Lyle 1987). Despite attempts in a number of authorities to operationalize this approach, translating the underlying concepts into a format for easy operational use remains problematic (Henwood et al. 1993). Nevertheless, as in the Social Services Inspectorate's (1993a) guidance on home support services, there is some indication of both a wish to incorporate these underlying principles into evaluation procedures and to tackle the issues this raises.

Within a health context, but with possible relevance to social care, is the development of a quality of life measure which allows subjects the freedom to choose the dimensions of most importance to them (McGee et al. 1991; O'Boyle et al. 1992). This measure is reportedly able to detect change over time, following some specified health interventions, but it is cumbersome to use and particularly difficult for people with any degree of cognitive impairment. Nevertheless, it may be further developed, and it illustrates that a greater degree of individualization of quality of life measures may be possible without losing the capacity to compare individuals and aggregate results.

In a different context, the Fife User Panels Project aims to establish whether membership of user panels leads to increased empowerment for older people (Cormie and Crichton 1994). The possibility of using existing measures (such as of self-esteem or life satisfaction) was rejected on the basis that they failed to explore the specific aspects of control and influence that underpinned the panels project. Instead, a questionnaire was designed to provide information about daily domestic life, support services, self-assertion and respect. The project consultant noted that the instrument lacks the 'apparent respectability of previous use' that may be associated with other measures, but argued that it addresses more specifically the questions raised within the project itself (ibid.: 17).

The existence of many studies or projects, trying different or related approaches, is to be welcomed. Once it is accepted that the perfect all-purpose measure for practice does not exist, there is a need and incentive to engage in, research and test a range of approaches. However, it becomes important to guard against fragmentation and duplication. There may be an important role for some central coordination to ensure that the existing knowledge is built upon, and that new lessons are shared and disseminated.

Implementing outcome measurement in routine practice

The links between research and practice

There is reason to doubt whether existing knowledge is effectively disseminated to or positively sought out by, practitioners: this applies both to the available measures and to knowledge about the likely outcomes of particular services. As noted in Chapter 1, commentators have argued that there is poor communication between the academic and practitioner communities, and a lack of a research culture among professionals and within SSDs: not only do social workers have no time to read at work, but to be seen doing so would imply that they do not have enough 'real' work (Fisher 1995). However, redefining research-based information as 'good practice', presenting it in readily digestible formats, and incorporating it into departmental guidelines and supervision procedures, can all help to make it more accessible to practitioners (Fisher 1995; Luker and Kenrick 1995).

As was discussed earlier, the introduction of outcome measurement needs to be based on clarity about the specific purpose of the exercise: whether the intention is, for example, to evaluate a specific service, to evaluate all services provided by one or several agencies, to monitor whether users' and carers' needs are being met, or to identify those services that achieve the 'best' outcomes for users and carers. These different purposes may require different approaches, some of which may not be achievable in routine practice.

Chapter 2 discussed a number of possible opportunities to incorporate outcome measurement for service users and carers into existing practice: the processes of assessment and review, inspection and contract monitoring are obvious examples (Box 9.3), which will be discussed further below. In some cases, routine outcome measurement may involve the collection of data about all people receiving services; in other instances, regular sampling may offer an opportunity to examine the impact of services. Focused studies, too, can become an integral part of departments' monitoring practice: they can be used to explore specific services in depth and from a variety of perspectives, and to identify and raise awareness about desirable outcomes.

Box 9.3   Potential organizational contexts for outcome measurement

- Care management assessments and reviews
- Inspection
- Contracting

The assessment and review process

Assessment and review processes seem to offer an obvious opportunity to incorporate ways of looking at outcomes. In theory at least, assessment provides a baseline against which later achievements can be checked at review. Following the implementation of the new community care arrangements, a great deal of attention has been given to the assessment process. It is acknowledged that monitoring and review have been traditionally 'under-resourced', and that local authorities tend to play down their importance compared with assessment and care planning (Social Services Inspectorate/NHSE 1994: 34). Our own research with a number of SSDs suggests that implementing review processes is seen as problematic. The volume of assessments generates considerable pressure of work so that review may be irregular or not carried out at all. Where reviews take place, they may simply consist of a check that the planned services are in fact being provided. In some cases review officers have been appointed but their main function may be to determine whether services could be withdrawn after a period of time. This is certainly an improvement over no review at all, but a failure to devote resources and attention to the review process represents a lost opportunity to examine in more detail whether service objectives have been achieved, and whether the services provided are in fact meeting the needs identified to the satisfaction of the service user or carer, and to the level that the SSD would expect.

Of course there may be some scepticism about the congruence between the model we have presented with what actually happens in practice. Do care plans in fact contain objectives? Is the recording of assessments sufficiently well undertaken to provide a baseline against which the results of any subsequent review can be checked? Such questions return us to issues of professional and organizational cultures and the degree to which a systematic consideration of outcomes can fit within these, or whether it requires culture change. Attempts to introduce changes in professional culture, such as the training of social workers in methods of single case evaluation, have met with some limited success (Kazi 1994) but, as we observed in Chapter 1, there is professional resistance to the specification and measurement of objectives, and evidence about the effectiveness of particular forms of social work practice seems to have had little impact (MacDonald *et al.* 1992).

Professional culture and implementing change

Some evidence is available about attempts to introduce more systematic monitoring and recording within social work and community care, and there is also a wider general literature on managing change in organizations. Together these suggest that the chances of successfully implementing the collection of outcome information will be increased if there is an understanding of the self-perceived needs and behaviour of those who are operating the system at the front line. As Lipsky (1980) pointed out, the necessary exercise of discretion by front-line professionals, and their relative autonomy from organizational authority, mean that more systematic performance measurement or monitoring procedures can be difficult if not impossible to implement. Any apparent attempt to challenge frontline professionals' practice may be subverted, or result in reduced morale and inhibit initiative: the mutual dependence of managers and front-line staff means that the introduction of accountability systems or measurement procedures requires a joint approach for its success, not the imposition of top–down procedures.

At present, many front-line professional staff are said to be resistant to further data collection (Oliver 1991; Priest and McCarthy 1993). Some feel that they already have insufficient time to cope with the demands being made of them, and that they should concentrate on providing a service to users rather than on extra paperwork (Hoyes *et al.* 1994). Such views may be reinforced by previous experiences of data collection that have not led to any change in practice or service provision. Other staff may see data collection solely as a means whereby management seeks to exert control over practitioners' work and professional standards: therefore a move to be resisted. The scepticism of staff about the real purposes of initiatives which purport to relate to quality may in some cases be justified: James (1994: 200) observes:

> . . . reflecting on how quality has been employed in public service organisation in the 1970s, 1980s and early 1990s would suggest that implementing quality has done little to improve services to users in practice . . . at . . . an early stage in formal development of quality in their departments, Social Services Departments were using it primarily

as a means of financial restraint, secondly as a demonstration of policy achievement, and only thirdly as a mechanism to enhance service to users.

In relation to outcome measurement, staff may be sceptical of the measures proposed, arguing that individual users have unique needs that cannot be encompassed within a standardized framework, or that good social work performance cannot necessarily be expressed in tangible, readily measurable outcomes (Carter 1988; Crompton and McMillan 1994). For others, the measures they are asked to apply may prove difficult to understand (Priest and McCarthy 1993). Such professional and practical concerns may lead to a call for systematic assessment and review of outcomes to become a component of professional training so that, rather than being undertaken explicitly with the aid of questionnaires and forms, it becomes an internalized part of professional practice, whereby professional staff both define and monitor outcomes as an integral part of their involvement with service users. This, in our view, would represent a means of improving practice, as well as offering a more compatible basis for the development of systems which would provide aggregated information.

One way of encouraging greater practitioner participation in evaluation is to allow operational staff to develop a sense of ownership of the process, rather than feeling it is being imposed on them (Priest and McCarthy 1993). This would, however, generate additional work and they would still need to be persuaded of its value: participation cannot be taken for granted. There is evidence, though, that staff have more positive attitudes towards monitoring systems which they have been involved in developing (Goldberg and Warburton 1979; Priest and McCarthy 1993), and that a participatory approach leads to the development of more relevant information systems. At the same time, a participatory approach to development is not enough: changed ways of working have to be supported by existing and continuing incentive structures if they are to be maintained (Mumford 1991). Incentives do not have to be financial: evidence suggests that changes are more likely to endure if they solve problems which are recognized by those who are involved in implementing the system, and if they fit well into existing professional value systems and practices (Domoney 1993). Tanenbaum (1994) noted that medical practitioners rely more on personal experience than on outcome data: however, they may use such data as a tool for practice if it is presented as complementary to their professional judgement, rather than seeking to replace it.

There is limited evidence about the introduction of formal review systems into social work. The study by Goldberg and Warburton (1979) involved a Case Review System (CRS) for use by social workers. Only one professional in the study criticized the system because the forms used did not give expression to the feelings and views of service users – though that study took place many years ago and more staff may consider this an important issue now. Although there was only a partial commitment to the CRS as an aid to individual practice, it did receive wider acceptance as a monitoring and planning tool that enabled social workers to compare their own practice with the work of colleagues. The study raised important issues about the extent to which the enthusiasm and commitment which may be engendered in staff who have been involved in creating and researching a monitoring instrument can be maintained when the same instrument is introduced across the board to staff who have played no such role. This is a theme which recurs in more recent literature (Philp *et al.* 1994). The latter study suggested that staff placed a greater value on the systematic collection of data which related to areas that were not normally well incorporated in their practice. Thus, staff in a secondary health care setting particularly valued information about relatives' stress levels and outcomes after discharge. Nevertheless, not all groups of staff proved able to incorporate additional data collection into their routine practice. Fletcher (1993) has suggested that, until staff are willing to gather the necessary data, there is no point in even starting to measure outcomes. Regular reviews may be promoted in terms of good professional practice (Social Services Inspectorate/ SWSG 1991), but this does not ensure they will be carried out (Priest and McCarthy 1993). Work is needed to identify those aspects of professional and organizational culture that might enhance or inhibit the routine collection of community care outcome data by frontline staff.

Self-assessment by users and carers

In some SSDs, the assessment process is essentially based on users' and carers' own definitions of needs. Where no 'objective' measures have been used initially, the subsequent measurement of outcomes will similarly have to follow a more user-based format. It may be that some users and carers would themselves like to collect outcome information. Experiments in self-assessment have suggested that willingness to undertake this may vary by user group: younger disabled people, for example, may be more interested in doing so than older people (personal communication from one SSD).

Aggregating data for management information

In addition to providing information which indicates how well services are meeting the needs of individual users – as well as possible needs for further support – the assessment and review process is also a potential source of information for management and planning purposes. One of the requirements is then for appropriate computer systems – and such systems are still far from well established in many SSDs (Social Services Inspectorate 1993). Research and information staff will also be needed to process and analyse the data: in many SSDs, the time of such staff is largely devoted to gathering demographic information and activity data, and possibly some survey work.

Some SSDs, nevertheless, are designing information systems which will record details of all assessments and, in some cases, outcomes too. The experiences of such authorities highlight the importance of working closely with practitioners to establish the value of such systems, rather than instituting complex additional procedures which practitioners may see as unnecessary bureaucratic impositions. Some systems, moreover, are being introduced on a interagency basis, specifically involving both health and social services: they show that it is possible to overcome the frequently mentioned difficulties associated with confidentiality and access by multiple agencies. While such systems offer a means of coordinating services for individual users, they also provide a source of information for interagency planning.

Inspection and audit

In some cases, it may not be appropriate for front-line staff to gather data themselves. This would apply, for instance, where outcome measurement is based on staff's subjective evaluations of the effectiveness of their own work. Users, for their part, may be unwilling to tell staff directly about any criticisms they may have. In such cases, outcomes may be more usefully assessed by an independent evaluator or inspector: users, of course, have an important role as service inspectors in their own right. Inspections which occur at only one point in time cannot directly collect outcome information, although they can ask some users or carers for their views about the effectiveness of services.

Nevertheless, the experience of the failure of inspection or accreditation visits to uncover serious abuse and neglect of people in institutions gives an indication of the limitations of such forms of evaluation. Felce (1986) cites a North American study in which researchers recorded an increase in staff activity with service users of over 200 per cent during an accreditation visit (Bible and Sneed 1976). In addition, there is reason to believe that the judgements of individual inspectors may not be as reliable as might be hoped. Gibbs and Sinclair (1992a) conducted a study designed to compare the ratings of residential facilities made independently by different inspectors. They argued that ratings of quality of care were best based on indicators of process rather than outcome, and they briefed inspectors in the use of a checklist based on the values of privacy, dignity, independence, rights, choice and fulfilment, as outlined in *Homes Are For Living In* (*HAFLI*) (Social Services Inspectorate 1989). Gibbs and Sinclair (1992b) observe that although it may be assumed that older people are unlikely to disagree with the values which underlie the *HAFLI* approach, it is not known how important these values are to them relative to others. The study looked at agreement between inspectors (making judgements independently) on a global six-point rating of quality, as well as agreement on the separate indicators which reflected the six key values. Levels of agreement were only 'slight', little better than chance, and considerably below what would be deemed acceptable as evidence in a tribunal. Such demonstrably unreliable measures of quality would provide little support for a purchaser in the event of any dispute with a residential care provider. One positive point to emerge from the research was that it did seem possible to reliably pick out homes of poor quality in the private sector. However, the authors concluded that it appeared to be very difficult to make reliable judgements on the quality of care in local authority homes using checklists (ibid.: 547). They also called for more research and development work in relation to the inspection process. If inspection focuses on process, what is needed is a firm basis in research which demonstrates that the aspects of process addressed are indeed related to better outcomes for individuals. Of course, periodic independent studies with a greater outcome focus might be carried out as an extension to the inspection process, or as another strand in quality assurance, or in relation to the monitoring of community care charters. Such studies might examine issues raised through the collection of quantitative data or as a means of exploring – and perhaps comparing – the impact of particular services.

Audit

Audit, for its part, is a cycle of activity which involves the systematic review of practice, development of possible improvements, implementation of these, and further review. The simplest distinction between audit and research is that research establishes the 'right thing' to do and audit investigates whether the right thing is being done. Audit does not necessarily involve outcome measurement, although it may do so. If research provides a basis for confidence that a particular type of intervention or service will produce the desired outcome, then it may be sufficient to review whether or not the activities of service providers are as prescribed. In situations where the connection between particular forms of service activity and definite outcomes for users is not well established, it would seem important to attempt to check actual outcomes against those believed to be being produced. Procedures for clinical audit are increasingly being introduced in health services and considerable resources have been made available for this – although a debate is still taking place about its overall impact and usefulness (Malby 1995). Unlike financial audit, it is generally carried out by staff involved in delivering services, although there may be outside assistance in developing and implementing the process. The introduction of a similar model of audit into social services would provide a potential area in which techniques for outcome measurement would be useful.

The contracting process

As was noted in Chapter 2, service contracts typically focus on activities and inputs rather than outcomes; or, if outcomes are referred to at all, it is in global terms that do not indicate how they might be monitored in practice. While an activity-based approach to contracting continues to be the norm, there are increasing moves towards an outcome-based approach. Osborne and Gaebler (1992) quote the example of nursing homes in the USA being rewarded for assisting people to regain independence rather than being paid more for residents who are confined to their beds. They note that an outcome-oriented approach is not only of greater benefit for individual users: it can help policymakers to know whether policies are succeeding or not.

Williams *et al.* (1993) describe the process of 'outcome funding' in more detail. This approach is based on the clear specification of performance targets: for instance, that a given percentage of users should increase their social contacts in a way that can be readily measured or observed. Once targets have been set, the means of achieving them can be specified (Marsden 1993); however, this, too, needs to be formulated in terms of users' activities or 'milestones', not inputs on the part of service providers. Purchasers of service, for their part, are seen as 'investors' wishing to purchase a particular product, rather than simply funding an activity. Providers' performance can itself be tied to payment: payments can be made contingent on achieving a specified result, or a lower fixed fee can be augmented by a bonus for higher-than-predicted performance. In addition to verification through achievement of the desired target outcomes, service effectiveness can be monitored by asking users about the changes they feel have occurred as a result of using the service. Williams *et al.* acknowledge that such verification, like the target setting itself, may lack scientific rigour. However, they note that investors often cannot afford, and may not need, a high degree of precision. Given that users are experts about the nature of their needs or problems, their views about service effectiveness are important. The use of more than one independent measure can help to verify what outcomes have been achieved.

Although the 'outcome funding' approach derives from public sector contracting with voluntary organizations in the USA, it is seen as an appropriate model for the new contracting arrangements for social care in the UK (Marsden 1993). Its most obvious applicability lies in the funding of projects for small groups of service users for whom a clear behaviour change is seen as desirable, as in the case of people with drug or alcohol problems. Nevertheless, it would appear to offer purchasers of social care services as a whole a means of shifting the focus of contracts from activities by service providers to outcomes for users.

The way forward

A good deal of work remains to be carried out, and a number of questions need to be addressed (see Box 9.4), if we are to deepen our understanding of the outcomes of community care and examine how outcome measurement might be incorporated into routine practice. It is, for example, unclear how broad principles – such as the promotion of independence – might be translated into measurable form, or how their measurement could be combined with aspects of outcomes that may only be applicable to some users. Further work will also be needed to establish whether a standardized approach to outcome measurement is possible, or whether it will always be necessary to examine individual users' circumstances and experiences in detail. We suspect that different approaches may be needed, depending on the purpose of measurement: for instance, whether it is part of the review process for individual users, or whether it is designed to assess the overall effectiveness of a service or to inform service planning. There are many opportunities to explore such issues: the field of community care is broad, and information about outcomes, and how to measure them, needs to be derived from many different contexts.

Box 9.4   The way forward: general questions

- What is the relative importance of – and relationship between – general service objectives and individual needs in determining outcomes?
- How feasible is it to adopt a standardized approach that allows for aggregation, as opposed to an approach that focuses on individual circumstances?
- What issues arise in the course of implementing outcome measurement in routine practice? How can problems be overcome?

Box 9.5 shows some of the steps that Social Services Departments and community health services might incorporate into the examination of outcomes. One important element in such work must be to consult users, carers and other stakeholders about service objectives and desirable outcomes. It will be necessary to establish how much consensus can be reached between them. The existing knowledge base about the impact of particular services and possible appropriate measures can then be drawn upon to inform the development and testing of outcome measures for use in routine practice. By aggregating the results of a number of more specific studies, it will be possible to determine which aspects of outcome are important to all users, and which may only be relevant to some. Once the possible domains have been identified, experimental work might build on models which allow users to select those domains that are important to them.

Box 9.5   Opportunities for developmental work by social services departments and community health services

- Identify an issue or service of particular concern
- Obtain users' and carers' views about desirable outcomes
- Translate policy objectives into outcomes for individuals
- Examine opportunities for involving both social and health care agencies
- Seek to establish consensus (or agreement to differ) between users, carers, professional staff and managers about desirable outcomes
- Refer to existing literature about outcomes of specific services and about methods of investigating particular dimensions of outcomes
- Design and test methods for determining whether outcomes have been achieved
- Measure inputs and seek to attribute outcomes to inputs

The difficulty of distinguishing between the outcomes of some health and social care services indicates that an interagency approach may often be desirable. This is most likely to be feasible where agencies are jointly commissioning a service: such a service may offer an appropriate starting point for joint outcome measurement. Where services are not being planned, purchased or provided jointly, the process of defining outcomes is likely to be more complex, and the process of implementing measurement on a routine basis even more so. Nevertheless, the importance for users and carers of an effective overall service – and the unimportance for them of agency boundaries – represent powerful incentives to adopt a joint approach.

If outcome measurement is to be incorporated into routine practice, the implementation process needs to be examined in detail. This involves the exploration of potential difficulties for practitioners responsible for gathering the necessary information, and of ways of ensuring that such information can either assist them in providing better services for individual users or provide useful feedback about the outcomes of services as a whole. There would appear to be a role for comparative experiments involving different assessment processes and different ways of collecting outcome information: for instance, structured, open-ended and user-led approaches. Opportunities to incorporate outcome measurement into inspection procedures, performance review, quality assurance or contracting also need to be explored. Not least, the possibilities of users measuring outcomes for themselves offer a valuable potential means of monitoring service effectiveness, provided users' feedback is properly acknowledged and not seen as a means of circumventing agency responsibilities.

Finally, there is a need to ensure that existing knowledge, about either outcome measures or the effectiveness of particular kinds of services, is more widely disseminated and used to inform planning and practice. At the same time, current knowledge about both effective dissemination procedures and the dynamics of organizational or professional change is very limited. The provision of information on its own is not enough: the environmental and cultural constraints that influence whether information leads to action need to be better understood.

Some caveats

Box 9.6   Warnings

- Outcome measurement should not focus only on what is most easily measurable
- Using broad categories may not identify specific outcomes
- Satisfaction surveys may not reveal anything about outcomes
- Involving practitioners in collecting information about outcomes may introduce certain kinds of bias
- Outcome measurement involves costs

Whatever approach is selected, it is important that the information that is gathered is not simply that which is most readily available (see Box 9.6): those aspects of a service or of outcomes that are easiest to measure may not be the most important ones. Using broad categories of needs (as often occurs in case review systems) may fail to clarify the precise nature or extent of those needs, and the impact of services that are subsequently provided may similarly be unclear. Focusing on satisfaction and dissatisfaction alone could divert attention from the evaluation of service effectiveness by not taking account of low expectations or a lack of information. A further danger is that agencies may examine those aspects of outcomes that are likely to reinforce their own values or beliefs; and practitioners can exercise bias in the way they complete evaluation schedules. Not least, the costs of operationalizing outcome measures have to be weighed against the potential benefits. Measures that are costly in terms of the time required for implementation or analysis, for instance, may carry high opportunity costs in relation to the direct services that could otherwise be provided for users and carers. Nevertheless, the very fact that resources are limited makes it desirable to provide the most cost-effective form of service available, for which information about outcomes is necessary.

Conclusions

This review does not offer any simple solutions to the task of outcome measurement. Its intention has been to clarify the conceptual, methodological and practical issues surrounding the collection of information about the impacts which services may have on those who receive them or are affected by them. We have given an overview of the existing knowledge base and indicated some possible ways forward for research and development. However, we recognize the danger in seeing outcome measurement on its own as a panacea for other policy or management problems (Hunter 1994). If such measurement is to inform the provision of more effective services, it is necessary to place it within the broader organizational context and not view it in isolation from factors such as professional culture, high workloads or resource limitations.

From our review of the field, we are led to conclude that future development work should proceed on the basis of four underlying principles:

- The existence of different stakeholders should be explicitly recognized and incorporated into the work.
- The views of service users and their carers are of key importance.
- Professional expertise and research-based knowledge are both useful in constructing measures.
- An understanding of the context in which the measures are to be implemented has an important bearing on their likely usefulness.

The possibilities for useful development work are many. While the difficulties should not be underestimated, nor should they be seen as a deterrent to further progress. Small-scale studies will not only add to the general understanding of outcomes and how to measure them: they can also be used to improve the specific services under examination.

The potential rewards are many. For agencies, outcome measurement offers an opportunity to ensure that their resources and efforts are used in the most effective way: it will provide evidence about their performance and a basis for purchasing and providing effective services. For front-line practitioners, it will indicate how well they are managing to meet users' needs and whether alternative or additional services are required. And, most importantly, it will offer users and carers a source of information about the impact of services, as well as a means of monitoring whether the services they receive are providing the support and assistance they require. Shifting the focus of monitoring towards outcomes will not be easy – but the benefits will justify the effort required.

Summary

A good deal of work has been undertaken on outcomes in health care, and some of this could inform outcome measurement in social care. Research on community care has also examined some aspects of outcomes for users and carers, though the instruments used have often been long and unsuitable for routine operational use. The development of more suitable measures or approaches, however, requires that attention be paid to a number of important issues:

- The measures have to reflect users' and carers' own definitions of appropriate community care outcomes. Users and carers have seldom been involved in the development of existing measures. However, if their views about needs and services are to underpin the new community care arrangements, it is essential that their views of outcomes should inform the evaluation of the impact of those services.
- Outcome measurement must take account of the specific objectives of the new arrangements, including independence, choice and personal control. Few existing measures examine such issues.
- There is a need to take account of the objections that may be raised by front-line staff to the gathering of further information. They may dispute its ability to effect policy changes or object to the additional time it could require – time which they can ill afford. Alternatively, they may perceive it as a management-inspired move to control their work and professional autonomy, or maintain that the impacts of their work are complex and cannot be readily measured. If routine outcome measurement requires their active participation, such resistances will need to be overcome.

While data collection by front-line staff offers one means of measuring outcomes through the assessment and review process, other organizational contexts also provide opportunities to examine outcomes of particular services. Inspection procedures can include a focus on outcomes, as can performance review and quality assurance. 'Outcome funding', for its part, offers a radical shift away from contracting based on activity by providers to outcomes for service users.

The lack of ready-made outcome measures, together with the complexity of community care, indicates a need for a wide range of studies and exploratory work by Social Services Departments, community health services and research units. The issues to be examined should include:

- users', carers' and other stakeholders' views about desirable outcomes;
- whether it is possible to achieve consensus between the different parties;
- establishing which aspects of community care would be applicable to all users, and which may only be relevant to some;

- investigating the problems of incorporating outcome measurement into routine practice;
- comparing the relative merits of different organizational contexts and procedures for measuring outcomes; and
- examining the way that existing knowledge about outcome measures or service effectiveness could be used to inform planning and professional practice.

REFERENCES

Ager, A. (1993) The life experiences checklist: part 2. Applications in service evaluation and quality assurance. *Mental Handicap*, 21: 46–48.

Aharony, L. and Strasser, S. (1993) Patient satisfaction: what we know about and what we still need to explore. *Medical Care Review*, 50(1): 49–79.

Alaszewski, A. and Manthorpe, J. (1993) Quality and the welfare services: a literature review. *British Journal of Social Work*, 23: 653–665.

Alison, V. and Wright, F. (1990) *Still Caring: a study of older parents still caring at home for a daughter or son with cerebral palsy.* London: The Spastics Society.

Allen, I., Hogg, D. and Peace, S. (1992) *Elderly People: choice, participation and satisfaction.* London: Policy Studies Institute.

Allen, D. and Lowe, K. (1995) Providing intensive community support to people with learning disabilities and challenging behaviour: a preliminary analysis of outcomes and costs. *Journal of Intellectual Disability Research*, 39: 67–82.

Anderson, R.T., Aaronson, N.K. and Wilkin, D. (1993) Critical review of the international assessments of health related quality of life. *Quality of Life Research*, 2: 369–395.

Arber, S., Gilbert, G.N. and Evandrou, M. (1988) Gender, household composition and receipt of domiciliary services by elderly disabled people. *Journal of Social Policy*, 17(2): 153–175.

Arnstein, S.R. (1969) A ladder of citizen participation. *Journal of the American Institute of Planners*, 35: 216–224.

Askham, J. and Thompson, C. (1990) *Dementia and Home Care: a research report on a home support scheme for dementia sufferers.* London: Age Concern.

Audit Commission (1992a) *Community Care: managing the cascade of change.* London: HMSO.

Audit Commission (1992b) *The Community Revolution: personal social services and community care.* London: HMSO.

Audit Commission (1992c) *Charting a Course.* London: HMSO.

Audit Commission (1993) *Staying on Course: the second year of the Citizen's Charter indicators*. London: HMSO.

Audit Commission (1994) *Watching their Figures: a guide to the Citizen's Charter indicators*. London: HMSO.

*Baldock, J. and Ungerson, C. (1994) *Becoming Consumers of Community Care: households within the mixed economy of welfare*. York: Joseph Rowntree Foundation.

Baldwin, S., Godfrey, C. and Propper, C. (eds) (1990) *Quality of Life: perspectives and policies*. London: Routledge.

Bardsley, M.J. and Coles, J.M. (1992) Practical experiences in auditing patient outcomes. *Quality in Health Care*, 1: 124–130.

Barnes, M. (1992) Beyond satisfaction surveys: involving people in research. *Generations Review*, 2(4): 15–17.

Barnes, M. and Miller, N. (eds) (1988) Performance measurement in personal social services. *Research, Policy and Planning*, 6(2): 1–47.

Barry, M.M., Crosby, C. and Mitchell, D.A. (1992) Quality of life issues in the evaluation of mental health services, in D.R. Trent (ed.), *Promotion of Mental Health*, Vol. 1. Aldershot: Avebury.

Beardshaw, V. (1988) *Last on the List: community services for people with physical disabilities*. London: King's Fund Institute.

Bebbington, A. and Quine, L. (1987) A comment on Hirst's 'Evaluating the Malaise Inventory'. *Social Psychiatry and Psychiatric Epidemiology*, 22: 5–7.

Becker, M., Diamond, R. and Sainfort, F. (1993) A new patient focused index for measuring quality of life in persons with severe and persistent mental illness. *Quality of Life Research*, 2(4): 239–251.

Beeforth, M., Conlan, E., Field, V., Hoser, B. and Sayce, L. (eds) (1990) *Whose Service is it Anyway? Users Views on Co-ordinating Community Care*. London: Research and Development for Psychiatry.

Bercovici, S. (1983) *Barriers to Normalisation: the restrictive management of retarded persons*. Baltimore, Maryland: University Park Press.

Beresford, B.A. (1994) *Positively Parents: caring for a severely disabled child*. SPRU Papers. London: HMSO.

Beresford, P. and Campbell, J. (1994) Disabled people, service users, user involvement and representation. *Disability and Society*, 9(3): 315–325.

Berger, M., Hill, P. and Walk, D. (1993) A suggested framework for outcomes in child and adolescent mental health services, in M. Berger, P. Hill, E. Sein, M. Thompson and C. Verduyn (eds) *Proposed Core Data Set for Child and Adolescent Psychology and Psychiatry Service*. London: Association for Child Psychology and Psychiatry.

Bergmann, K., Gaber, L.B. and Foster, E.M. (1975) The development of an instrument for early ascertainment of psychiatric disorder in elderly community residents: A pilot study. *Gerontopsychiatric*, 4: 84–119.

Berry, L.L., Zeithaml, V.A. and Parasuraman, A. (1985) Quality counts in service too. *Business Horizons*, 28(3): 44–52.

Beswick, J., Zadik, T. and Felce, D. (eds) (1986) *Evaluating Quality of Care*. Conference series. Kidderminster: British Institute of Mental Handicap.

Bewley, C. and Glendinning, C. (1994) *Involving Disabled People in Community Care Planning*. York: Joseph Rowntree Foundation.

Bible, G.H. and Sneed, T.J. (1976) Some effects of an accreditation survey on program completion at a state institution. *Mental Retardation*, 14: 14–15.

Bird, A.S., MacDonald, A.J.D., Mann, A.H. and Philpott, M.P. (1987) Preliminary experience with the selfcare (D): a self-rating depression questionnaire for use in elderly, non-institutionalised subjects. *International Journal of Geriatric Psychiatry*, 2: 31–38.

Blyth, A. (1990) Audit of terminal care in a general practice. *British Medical Journal*, 300: 983–986.

Bond, S. (1992) *Outcomes of Nursing: proceedings of an institutional developmental workshop*. Newcastle upon Tyne: Centre for Health Service Research, University of Newcastle upon Tyne.

Booth, T., Simons, K. and Booth, W. (1990) *Outward Bound: relocation and community care for people with learning difficulties*. Buckingham: Open University Press.

Bowling, A. (1991) *Measuring Health: a review of quality of life measurement scales*. Buckingham: Open University Press.

Bowling, A. (1995) *Measuring Disease: a review of disease-specific quality of life measurement scales*. Buckingham: Open University Press.

Bradshaw, J.R. and Lawton, D. (1978) Tracing the causes of stress in families with handicapped children. *British Journal of Social Work*, 8: 181–192.

Brazier, J.E., Harper, R., Jones, N.M.B., O'Cathain, A., Thomas, K.J., Usherwood, T. and Westlake, L. (1992) Validating the SF-36 health survey questionnaire: new outcome measure for primary care. *British Medical Journal*, 305: 160–164.

Bristol Advocacy Project (1993) Citizen advocacy and people with learning difficulties. *Social Care Research Findings*, No. 42. York: Joseph Rowntree Foundation.

Brown, H. and Smith, H. (1992) *Normalisation: a reader for the nineties*. London: Tavistock/Routledge.

Burningham, D. (1990) Performance indicators and the management of professionals in local government, in M. Cave, M. Kogan, and R. Smith (eds) *Output and Performance Measurement in Government: the state of the art*. London: Jessica Kingsley.

Burns, T., Beadsmoore, A., Bhat, A.V., Oliver, A. and Mathers, C. (1993) A controlled trial of home-based acute psychiatric services: clinical and social outcome. *British Journal of Psychiatry*, 163: 49–54.

Butler, K. and Forrest, A. (1990) Citizen advocacy for people with disabilities, in L. Winn (ed.) *Power to the People: the key to responsive services in health and social care*. London: King's Fund Centre.

Byrne, E.A. and Cunningham, C.C. (1985) The effects of mentally handicapped children on families – a conceptual review. *Journal of Child Psychology and Psychiatry*, 26(6): 847–864.

Cale, L. (1993) Information: the tool that enables, in *National Disability Information Project, Information Enables: improving access to information services for disabled people*. London: Policy Studies Institute.

Calnan, M. (1988) Towards a conceptual framework of lay evaluation of health care. *Social Science and Medicine*, 27(9): 927–933.

Campbell, P. (1990) Mental health self-advocacy, in L. Winn (ed.) *Power to the*

People: the key to responsive services in health and social care. London: King's Fund Centre.

Cambridge P., Knapp M. and Hayes, L. (1991) *Framework Paper: methodologies and hypotheses for evaluating long-term outcomes and costs of care in the community for people with learning difficulties, DP 705.* Canterbury: PSSRU, University of Kent.

⊛Carers' Alliance (undated) *A Carers' Manifesto.* London: Carers' Alliance.

Carr-Hill, R. (1992) The measurement of patient satisfaction. *Journal of Public Health Medicine,* 14(3): 236–249.

Carr-Hill, R., Dixon, P. and Thompson, A. (1989) Too simple for words. *Health Service Journal,* 15 June 1989: 728–729.

Carter, R.D. (1988) Measuring client outcomes: the experience of the States. *Administration in Social Work,* 11(3/4): 73–88.

Cartwright, A. and Seale, C. (1990) *The Natural History of a Survey: an account of the methodological issues encountered in a study of life before death.* London, King's Fund Centre.

Centre for Policy on Ageing (1990) *Community Life: a code of practice for community care.* London: CPA.

Challis, D.J. (1981) The measurement of outcome in social care of the elderly. *Journal of Social Policy,* 10(2): 179–208.

Challis, D. and Knapp, M. (1980) *An Examination of the PGC Morale Scale in an English Context.* PSSRU Discussion Paper 168. Canterbury: University of Kent.

Challis, D. and Davies, B. (1986) *Case Management in Community Care: an evaluated experiment in the home care of the elderly.* Aldershot: Gower.

Challis, D., Chessum, R., Chesterman, J., Luckett, R. and Traske, K. (1990) *Case Management in Social and Health Care.* Canterbury: PSSRU, University of Kent.

Charlton, J.R.H. (1989) Approaches to assessing disability, in D.L. Patrick, and H. Peach (eds) *Disablement in the Community.* Oxford: Oxford University Press.

Cheetham, J., Fuller, R., McIvor, G. and Petch, A. (1992) *Evaluating Social Work Effectiveness.* Buckingham: Open University Press.

Coleman, P.G. (1984) Assessing self-esteem and its sources in elderly people. *Ageing and Society,* 4: 117–135.

Common, R. and Flynn, N. (1992) *Contracting for Care.* York: Joseph Rowntree Foundation.

Conneally, S., Boyle, G. and Smyth, F. (1992) An evaluation of the use of small group homes for adults with a severe and profound mental handicap. *Mental Handicap Research,* 5(2): 146–187.

Copeland, J.R.M., Kelleher, M.J., Kellett, J.M., Gourlay, A.J., Gurland, B.J., Fleiss, J.L. and Sharpe, L. (1976) A semi-structural clinical interview for the assessment of diagnosis and mental state in the elderly: the geriatric mental state schedule. *Psychological Medicine,* 6: 439–449.

Connelly, N. (1990) *Raising Voices: Social Services Departments and people with disabilities.* London: Policy Studies Institute.

Cormie, J. and Crichton, M. (1994) *Fife User Panels Project: new ways of working.* Edinburgh: Age Concern Scotland.

Cox, E. and Parsons, R. (1994) *Empowerment-Oriented Social Work Practice with the Elderly.* Pacific Grove, California: Brooks/Cole.

⊁Creer, C., Sturt, E. and Wykes, T. (1982) The role of relatives, in J.K. Wing (ed.)

Long-term community care: experience in a London Borough. *Psychological Medicine*, Monograph Supplement 2, pp. 29–39. Cambridge: Cambridge University Press.

Croft, S. and Beresford, P. (1990) User involvement in the provision of services. *Social Care Research Findings*, No. 9. York: Joseph Rowntree Foundation.

Croft, S. and Beresford, P. (1993) *Getting Involved: a practical manual*. London: Open Services Project.

Crompton, T. and McMillan, C. (1994) Going places. *Community Care*, 10 March 1994: 28–29.

Crosby, C. and Barry, M.M. (eds) (1995) *Community Care: evaluation of the provision of mental health services*. Aldershot: Avebury.

Culyer, T. (1990) Commodities, characteristics of commodities, characteristics of people, utilities, and the quality of life, in S. Baldwin, C. Godfrey and C. Propper (eds) *Quality of Life: perspectives and policies*. London: Routledge.

Cunningham, C., Sloper, P. and Rangecroft, A. (1986) *Effects of Early Intervention on the Occurrence and Nature of Behaviour Problems in Children with Down's Syndrome. Report to DHSS*. Hester Adrian Research Centre, University of Manchester.

Dant, T., Carley, M., Gearing, B. and Johnson, M. (1989) *Care for Elderly People at Home: final report*. Milton Keynes: Open University/Policy Studies Institute.

Davies, B. and Challis, D. (1986) *Matching Resources to Needs in Community Care*. Aldershot, Gower.

Davies, B., Bebbington, A. and Charnley, H. (1990) *Resources Needs and Outcomes in Community-based Care: a comparative study of the production of welfare for elderly people in ten local authorities in England and Wales*. Aldershot: Avebury.

Davies, H. (1987) Performance measurement in local government, in NCC *Performance Measurement and the Consumer*. London: National Consumer Council.

de Jong, G. (1981) *Environmental Accessibility and Independent Living Outcomes: directions for disability policy and research*. University Center for International Rehabilitation: Michigan State University.

de Kock U., Saxby, H., Thomas, M. and Felce, D. (1988) Community and family contact: an evaluation of small community homes for adults. *Mental Handicap Research*, 1: 127–140.

Denham, M.J. and Jeffreys, P.M. (1972) Routine mental assessment in elderly patients. *Modern Geriatrics*, 2, 275.

Department of Health (1990) *Community Care in the Next Decade and Beyond: policy guidance*. London: HMSO.

Department of Health (1993) *Population Needs Assessment: good practice guidance*. London: Department of Health.

Department of Health (1994) *Monitoring and Development. First Impressions, April–September 1993*. London: Department of Health.

Department of Health and Social Security (1983) *Care in the Community and Joint Finance*. Health Circular HC(83)6. London: DHSS.

Domoney, L. (1993) *The Management of Innovations: literature review*. London: National Institute for Social Work.

Donabedian, A. (1992) Quality assurance in health care: consumers' role. *Quality in Health Care*, 1: 247–251.

Donnelly, M., McGilloway, S., Mays, N., Perry, S., Knapp, M., Kavanagh, S., Beecham, J., Fenyo, A. and Astin, J. (1994) *Opening New Doors: an evaluation of community care for people discharged from psychiatric and mental handicap hospitals*. London: HMSO.

Eagles, J.M., Craig, A., Rawlinson, F., Restall, D.B., Beattie, J.A.G. and Besson, J.A.O. (1987) The psychological well-being of supporters of the demented elderly. *British Journal of Psychiatry*, 150: 293–298.

Eakin, P. (1989a) Assessment of activities of daily living: a critical review. *British Journal of Occupational Therapy*, 52(1): 11–15.

Eakin, P. (1989b) Problems with assessments of activities of daily living. *British Journal of Occupational Therapy*, 52(2): 50–54.

Eddy, D.M. (1990) Comparing benefits and harms: the balance sheet. *Journal of the American Medical Association*, 263(18): 2493–2505.

Ellis, K. (1993) *Squaring the Circle: user and carer participation in needs assessment*. York: Joseph Rowntree Foundation.

Emerson, E. and Hatton, C. (1994) *Moving Out: relocation from hospital to community*. London: HMSO.

Emerson E., Mansell J. and McGill P. (eds) (1994) *Severe Learning Disabilities and Challenging Behaviours: designing high quality services*. London: Chapman and Hall.

Evans G. and Gray P. (1990) *Service Review Package*. Cardiff: Opportunity Housing Trust.

Evans, G., Todd, S., Beyer, S., Felce, D. and Perry, J. (1994) Assessing the impact of the All Wales mental handicap strategy: a survey of four districts. *Journal of Intellectual Disability Research*, 38: 109–33.

Fadden, G., Bebbington, P. and Kuipers, L. (1987) Caring and its burdens: a study of the spouses of depressed patients. *British Journal of Psychiatry*, 151: 660–667.

Fallowfield, L. (1990) *The Quality of Life: the missing measurement in health care*. London: Souvenir Press.

Felce, D. (1986) Evaluation by direct observation, in J. Beswick, T. Zadik and D. Felce (eds) *Evaluating Quality of Care*. Conference series. Kidderminster: British Institute of Mental Handicap.

Felce, D. and Perry, C. (1995) Quality of life: its definition and measurement. *Research in Developmental Disabilities*, 16(4): 51–74.

Felce, D., Thomas, M., de Kock, U., Saxby, H. and Repp, A. (1985) An ecological comparison of small community-based houses and traditional institutions for severely and profoundly mentally handicapped adults: II. Physical settings and use of opportunities. *Behaviour Research and Therapy*, 23, 337–348.

Fiedler, B. (1991) *Tracking Success: testing services for people with severe physical and sensory disabilities*. Living Options in Practice: Project Paper No. 2. London: King's Fund Centre.

Fiedler, B. (1993) *Getting Results: unlocking community care in partnership with disabled people*. Living Options Partnership: Paper No. 1. London: King's Fund Centre.

Fiedler, B. and Twitchin, D. (1992) *Achieving User Participation: planning services for people with severe physical and sensory disabilities*. Living Options in Practice: Project Paper No. 3. London: King's Fund Centre.

158   References

Fisher, M. (1983) The meaning of client satisfaction, in M. Fisher (ed.) *Speaking of Clients*. Social Services Monographs. Sheffield: Joint Unit for Social Services Research, University of Sheffield.

Fisher, T. (1995) A systematic knowledge base in child protection: what knowledge do social workers use? Mimeo. York: Department of Social Policy and Social Work, University of York.

Fitzpatrick, R. (1991) Surveys of patient satisfaction: important general considerations. *British Medical Journal*, 302: 887–889.

Fitzpatrick, R., Fletcher, A., Gore, S., Jones, D., Spiegelhalter, D. and Cox, D. (1992a) Quality of life measures in health care: applications and issues in assessment. *British Medical Journal*, 305: 1074–1077.

Fitzpatrick, R., Ziebland, S., Jenkinson, C., Mowat, A. and Mowat, A. (1992b) Importance of sensitivity to change as a criterion for selecting health status measures. *Quality in Health Care*, 1: 89–93.

Fletcher, A. (1993) Presentation at Health Outcomes '93 Conference, London, September, reported in R. MacLachlan and D. Glasman, A case of myth management. *Health Service Journal*, 16 September 1993: 12–13.

Fletcher, A.E., Dickinson, E.J. and Philp, I. (1992) Review. Audit measures: quality of life instruments for everyday use with elderly patients. *Age and Ageing*, 21: 142–150.

Flynn, M. (1986) Adults who are mentally handicapped as consumers: issues and guidelines for interviewing. *Journal of Mental Deficiency Research*, 30: 369–377.

Foulds, G.A. and Bedford, A. (1979) *Manual of the Delusions, Symptoms State Inventory*. Windsor: NFER.

Frater, A. (1992) Health outcomes: a challenge to the status quo. *Quality in Health Care*, 1: 87–88.

Fricke, J. (1993) Measuring outcomes in rehabilitation: a review. *British Journal of Occupational Therapy*, 56(6): 217–221.

Garratt, A.M., Ruta, D.A., Abdalla, M.I., Buckingham, J.K. and Russell, I.T. (1993) The SF36 health survey questionnaire: an outcome measure suitable for routine use within the NHS? *British Medical Journal*, 306: 1440–1444.

Gaster, L. (1991) *Quality at the Front Line*. Bristol: School of Advanced Urban Studies, University of Bristol.

Gaster, L. (1995) *Quality in Public Services: managers' choices*. Buckingham: Open University Press.

Gibbons, J.S., Horn, S.H., Powell, J.M. and Gibbons, J.L. (1984) Schizophrenic patients and their families: a survey in a psychiatric service based on a DGH unit. *British Journal of Psychiatry*, 144: 70–77.

Gibbs, I. and Sinclair, I. (1992a) Consistency: a prerequisite for inspecting old people's homes? *British Journal of Social Work*, 22, 535–550.

Gibbs, I. and Sinclair, I. (1992b) Checklists: their possible contribution to inspection and quality assurance in elderly people's homes, in D. Kelly and B. Warr (eds) *Quality Counts*. London: Whiting and Birch.

Gilhooly, M.L.M. (1984) The impact of care-giving on care-givers: factors associated with the psychological well-being of people supporting a dementing relative in the community. *British Journal of Medical Psychology*, 57: 35–44.

Gilleard, C.J. (1984) *Living with Dementia*. London: Croom Helm.

Gilleard, C.J. (1987) Influence of emotional distress among supporters on the outcome of psychogeriatric day care. *British Journal of Psychiatry*, 150: 219–223.

Gilleard, C.J., Belford, H., Gilleard, E., Whittick, J.E. and Gledhill, K. (1984) Emotional distress amongst the supporters of the elderly mentally infirm. *British Journal of Psychiatry*, 145: 172–177.

Goldberg, D.P. (1972) *The Detection of Psychiatric Illness by Questionnaire*. Maudsley Monograph No. 21. London: Oxford University Press.

Goldberg, E.M. and Warburton, R.W. (1979) *Ends and Means in Social Work: the development and outcome of a case review system for social workers*. Social Services Library No. 35. London: National Institute for Social Work.

Goldberg, E.M. and Connelly, N. (1982) *The Effectiveness of Social Care for the Elderly: an overview of recent and current evaluative research*. London: Heinemann Educational.

Goss, S. and Miller, C. (1993) *Initiatives in User and Carer Involvement: a survey of local authorities*. London: Office for Public Management.

Goss, S. and Miller, C. (1995) *From Margin to Mainstream: developing user- and carer-centred community care*. York: Joseph Rowntree Foundation/Community Care.

Grad, J. and Sainsbury, P. (1963) Mental illness and the family. *Lancet*, i: 544–547.

Grad, J. and Sainsbury, P. (1968) The effects that patients have on their families in a community care and a control psychiatric service – a two-year follow-up. *British Journal of Psychiatry*, 114: 265–278.

Grant, G. (1992) Researching user and carer involvement in mental handicap services, in M. Barnes and G. Wistow (eds) *Researching User Involvement*. Leeds: Nuffield Institute for Health Service Studies.

Grant, G. and Nolan, M. (1993) Informal carers: sources and concomitants of satisfaction. *Health and Social Care in the Community*, 1(3): 147–160.

Green, S. (1992) *Measuring Outcomes in the Mental Health Services*. Discussion Paper 29. Birmingham: Health Services Management Centre, University of Birmingham.

Greene, J.G., Smith, R., Gardiner, M. and Timbury, G.C. (1982) Measuring behavioural disturbance of elderly demented patients in the community and its effect on relatives: a factor analytic study. *Age and Ageing*, 11: 121–126.

Greenwood, R. and McMillan, T. (1993) An investigation into the effects of case-management after severe head injury, in D. Robbins (ed.) *Community Care: findings from Department of Health funded research 1988–1992*, pp. 354–357. London: HMSO.

Gregson, B. and Dawson, P. (1993) Adult community physiotherapy project, in D. Robbins (ed.) *Community Care: findings from Department of Health funded research 1988–1992*, pp. 341–342. London: HMSO.

Greveson, G. and James, O. (1991) Improving long-term outcome after stroke: the views of patients and carers. *Health Trends*, 23(4): 161–162.

Gurland, B. (1980) The assessment of mental health status in older adults, in J. Birren and R. Sloan (eds) *Handbook of Mental Health and Ageing*, pp. 671–700. New York: McGraw-Hill.

Hall, J.A., Roter, D.L. and Katz, N.R. (1988) Meta-analysis of correlates of provider behaviour in medical encounters. *Medical Care*, 26(7): 657–675.

*Harding, T. and Beresford, P. (1995) *What Service Users and Carers Value and Expect from Social Services Staff.* NISW/Open Services Project, Report to Department of Health.

Hardy, B., Wistow, G. and Leedham, I. (1993) *Analysis of a Sample of English Community Care Plans 1993/94.* Leeds: Nuffield Institute for Health.

Harries, U. and Hill, S. (1994) Two sides of the coin. *Health Service Journal*, 22 September 1994: 25.

Harrison, T. (1993) Commentary on 'Performance indicators: what was all the fuss about?' *Community Care Management and Planning*, 1(4): 99–105.

Heal, L. and Chadsey-Rusch, J. (1985) The Lifestyle Satisfaction Scale (LSS): assessing individuals' satisfaction with residence, community setting, and associated services. *Applied Research in Mental Retardation*, 6: 475–490.

Healy, M. and Potter, J. (1987) Making performance measurement work for consumers, in NCC *Performance Measurement and the Consumer.* London: National Consumer Council.

Henderson, S., Duncan-Jones, P., Byrne, D.G. and Scott, R. (1980) Measuring social relationships: the Interview Schedule for Social Interaction. *Psychological Medicine*, 10: 723–734.

Henwood, M. with Vyvyan, C. and Renshaw, J. (1993) *Measuring up to the Strategy? Learning Difficulties, Quality and the All Wales Strategy.* Cardiff: Welsh Office and Audit Commission.

Higginson I. (1994) Clinical teams, general practice, audit and outcomes, in T. Delamothe (ed.) *Outcomes into Clinical Practice.* London: BMJ Publishing Group.

Higginson, I., Wade, A. and McCarthy, M. (1990) Palliative care: views of patients and their families. *British Medical Journal*, 301: 277–281.

Hill, S. and Harries, U. (1993) The outcomes process: some reflections from research with people in their 60s and 70s. *Critical Public Health*, 4(4): 21–28.

Hill, S., Harries, U. and Popay, J. (1994) Assessing the Outcomes of Community Based Health Services for Older People: The Short Form 36's Responsiveness to Change. Draft manuscript. Public Health Research and Resource Centre, Salford.

Hirschman, A. (1970) *Exit, Voice and Loyalty: responses to decline in firms, organisations and states.* Harvard: Harvard University Press.

Hirst, M.A. (1983) Evaluating the Malaise Inventory: an item analysis. *Social Psychiatry*, 18: 181–184.

Hirst, M.A. and Bradshaw, J.R. (1983) Evaluating the Malaise Inventory: a comparison of measures of stress. *Journal of Psychosomatic Research*, 27(3): 193–199.

Hirst, M.A and Baldwin, S. (1994) *Unequal Opportunities: growing up disabled.* SPRU Papers. London: HMSO.

Hoenig, J. and Hamilton, M.W. (1969) *The Desegregation of the Mentally Ill.* London: Routledge and Kegan Paul.

Hogg, J. and Raynes, N. (eds) (1986) *Assessment in Mental Handicap: a guide to assessment practices, tests and checklists.* London: Chapman and Hall.

Holmes, N., Shah, A. and Wing, L. (1982) The Disability Assessment Schedule:

a brief screening device for use with the mentally retarded. *Psychological Medicine*, 12: 879–890.

House of Commons (1993) *Community Care: the way forward*, 6th Report of the Health Committee, HC 482-I. London: HMSO.

Hoyes, L. and Lart, R. (1992) Taking care. *Community Care*, 20 August 1992: 14–15.

Hoyes, L., Means, R. and Le Grand, J. (1992) *Made to Measure? Performance Measurement and Community Care*. Occasional Paper 39. School for Advanced Urban Studies. Bristol: University of Bristol.

Hoyes, L., Jeffers, S., Lart, R., Means, R. and Taylor, M. (1993) *User Empowerment and the Reform of Community Care*. Bristol: School for Advanced Urban Studies.

Hoyes, L., Means, R., Lart, R. and Taylor, M. (1994) *Community Care in Transition*. York: Joseph Rowntree Foundation.

Hughes, B. (1990) Quality of life, in S. Peace (ed.) *Researching Social Gerontology*. London: Sage.

Hughes, B. (1993) A model for the comprehensive assessment of older people and their carers. *British Journal of Social Work*, 23: 345–364.

Hughes, B. (1995) *Older People and Community Care: critical theory and practice*. Buckingham: Open University Press.

Hunter, D. (1994) Are we being effective? *Health Service Journal*, 16 June 1994: 23.

Huxley, P. and Mohamad, H. (1991) The development of a general satisfaction questionnaire for use in programme evaluation. *Social Work and Social Sciences Review*, 3(1): 63–74.

Independent Review Group (1994) *A Wider Strategy for Research and Development relating to Personal Social Services*. Report to Director of Research and Development, Department of Health. London: HMSO.

Israel, L., Kozarevic, D. and Sartorius, N. (1984) *Source Book of Geriatric Assessment*, Vol. 1 and Vol. 2. Basel: Karger.

James, A. (1992) Quality and its social construction by managers in care service organisations, in D. Kelly, and B. Warr, (eds) *Quality Counts: achieving quality in social care services*. London: Whiting and Birch.

James, A. (1993) Talking across boundaries. *Community Care*, Supplement, 27 May 1993: i–ii.

James, A. (1994) Reflections on the politics of quality, in A. Connor and S. Black (eds) *Performance Review and Quality in Social Care*. London: Jessica Kingsley.

James, A., with Brooks, T. and Towell, D. (1992) *Committed to Quality: quality assurance in Social Services Departments*. London: HMSO.

Jeffrey, L.I.H. (1993) Aspects of selecting outcome measures to demonstrate the effectiveness of comprehensive rehabilitation. *British Journal of Occupational Therapy*, 56(11): 394–400.

Jenkinson, C., Coulter, A. and Wright, L. (1993) Short Form 36 (SF36) health survey questionnaire: normative data for adults of working age. *British Medical Journal*, 306: 1437–1440.

Jowell, T. (1991) *Challenges and Opportunities*. Paper to Ministerial 'Policy and Practice' Conference, January 1991, distributed with *Caring for People Newsletter*, No. 4. London: Department of Health.

Judge, K. and Solomon, M. (1993) Public opinion and the National Health Service: patterns and perspectives in consumer satisfaction. *Journal of Social Policy*, 22(3): 299–327.

Kane, R.A. and Kane, R.L. (1981) *Assessing the Elderly: a practical guide to measurement*. Lexington: Lexington Books.

Kazi, M. (1994) Single Case Evaluation in Improving Services. Paper given at Association of Directors of Social Services National Research Conference, Stafford, November.

Keady, J. and Nolan, M. (1994) The Carer-Led Assessment Process (CLASP): a framework for the assessment of need in dementia caregivers. *Journal of Clinical Nursing*, 3: 103–108.

Kearney, P. and Miller, D. (1994) The numbers game. *Community Care*, 13 January 1994: 22–23.

Keep, J. and Clarkson, J. (1994) *Disabled People Have Rights: final report on a two-year project funded by the Nuffield Provincial Hospitals Trust*. London: The Royal Association for Disability and Rehabilitation.

Kemp, J. and Middleton, L. (1993) Personal packages. *Care Weekly*, 24 June 1993: 12.

Kernan, K. and Sabsay, S. (1984) Getting there: directions given by retarded and non-retarded adults, in R. Edgerton (ed.) *Lives in Process: mildly retarded adults in a large city*. Monograph No. 6. Washington DC: American Association on Mental Deficiency.

Kestenbaum, A. (1993) *Making Community Care a Reality: the Independent Living Fund 1988–1993*. Nottingham: Independent Living Fund.

Kind, P. (1990) Issues in the design and construction of a quality of life measure, in S. Baldwin, C. Godfrey and C. Propper (eds) *Quality of Life: perspectives and Policies*. London: Routledge.

King's Fund (1988) *Action for Carers: a guide to multi-disciplinary support at local level*. London: King's Fund Centre.

Knapp, M. (1984) *The Economics of Social Care*. Basingstoke: Macmillan.

Knapp, M., Cambridge, P., Thomason, C., Beecham, J., Allen, C. and Darton, R. (1992) *Care in the Community: challenge and demonstration*. Aldershot: Ashgate.

Kuriansky, J., Gurland, B. and Fliess, J. (1976) The assessment of self-care capacity in geriatric psychiatric patients by objective and subjective methods. *Journal of Clinical Psychology*, 32: 95–102.

Lakhani, A. (1992) Nursing outcomes research: a Department of Health perspective, in S. Bond (ed.) *Outcomes of Nursing: proceedings of an invitational workshop*. Newcastle upon Tyne: Centre for Health Services Research, University of Newcastle upon Tyne.

Lamb, B. and Layzell, S. (1994) *Disabled in Britain: a world apart*. London: Scope.

Landesman, S. (1987) The changing structure and function of institutions; a search for optimal group care environments, in S. Landesman and P. Vietze (eds) *Living Environments and Mental Retardation*. Washington DC: American Association on Mental Deficiency.

Lawton, M.P. (1975) The Philadelphia geriatric centre morale scale: a revision. *Journal of Gerontology*, 30: 85–89.

Lawton, M.P., Brody, E.M. and Saperstein, A.R. (1989) A controlled study of respite service for caregivers of Alzheimer's patients. *The Gerontologist*, 29(1): 8–16.

Leatherbarrow, M. (1994) Presentation at SSRG Workshop: 'Performance in Social Services: Potential and Realities', Birmingham, 28 January 1994.

Leckie, T. (1994) Quality assurance in social work, in A. Connor and S. Black (eds) *Performance Review and Quality in Social Care*. London: Jessica Kingsley.

Leedham, I. (1989) From mental handicap hospital to community provision. PhD Thesis, University of Kent.

Lehman, A.F., Ward, N.C. and Linn, L.S. (1982) Chronic mental patients: the quality of life issue, *American Journal of Psychiatry*, 139(10): 1271–1276.

Levin, E., Sinclair, I. and Gorbach, P. (1985) The effectiveness of the home help service with confused old people and their families. *Research, Policy and Planning*, 3(2): 1–7.

Levin, E., Sinclair, I. and Gorbach, P. (1989) *Families, Services and Confusion in Old Age*. Aldershot: Avebury.

Lewis, J. and Meredith, B. (1989) Contested territory in informal care, in M. Jefferys (ed.) *Growing Old in the Twentieth Century*, pp. 186–200. London: Routledge.

Linder-Pelz, S. (1982) Social psychological determinants of patient satisfaction: a test of five hypotheses. *Social Science and Medicine*, 16: 583–589.

Lipsky, M. (1980) *Street-Level Bureaucracy: dilemmas of the individual in public services*. New York: Russell Sage Foundation.

Locker, D. and Dunt, D. (1978) Theoretical and methodological issues in sociological studies of consumer satisfaction with medical care. *Social Science and Medicine*, 12: 283–292.

Lohr, K.N. (1988) Outcome measurement: concepts and questions. *Inquiry*, 25: 37–50.

Lohr, K.N. (1992) Applications of health status assessment measures in clinical practice: overview of the third conference on advances in health status measurement. *Medical Care*, 30(5), supplement: MS1–MS14.

London Research Centre (1991) *Support for Carers: carers' views on services*. London: LRC.

Luker, K.A. and Kenrick, M. (1995) Towards knowledge based practice: an evaluation of a method of dissemination, *International Journal of Nursing Studies*, 32(1): 59–67.

MacCarthy, B., Lesage, A., Brewin, C.R., Brugha, T.S., Mangen, S. and Wing, J.K. (1989) Needs for care among the relatives of long-term users of day care: a report from the Camberwell High Contact Survey. *Psychological Medicine*, 19: 725–736.

McConkey, R., Walsh, P. and Conneally, S. (1993) Neighbours' reactions to community services: contrasts before and after services open in their locality. *Mental Handicap Research*, 6: 131–141.

McCreadie, R.G., Crocket, G.T., Livingston, M.G., Todd, N.A., Loudon, J., Batchelor, D. and Menzies, C.W. (1987) The Scottish first episode schizophrenia study. IV. Psychiatric and social impact on relatives. *British Journal of Psychiatry*, 150: 340–344.

MacDonald, G. and Sheldon, B. with Gillespie, J. (1992) Contemporary studies of the effectiveness of social work. *British Journal of Social Work*, 22(6): 615–643.

McDowell, I. and Newell, C. (1987) *Measuring Health: a guide to rating scales and questionnaires.* Oxford: Oxford University Press.

McGee, H., O'Boyle, C., Hickey, A., O'Malley K. and Joyce, C. (1991) Assessing the quality of life of the individual: SEIQoL with a healthy and a gastroenterology unit population. *Psychological Medicine,* 21, 749–759.

McGill, P., Emerson, E. and Mansell, J. (1994) Individually designed residential provision for people with seriously challenging behaviours, in E. Emerson, J. Mansell and P. McGill (eds) *Severe Learning Disabilities and Challenging Behaviours: designing high quality services.* London: Chapman and Hall.

MacGuire, J. (1990) Putting Nursing Research Findings into practice: research utilisation as an aspect of the management of change. *Journal of Advanced Nursing,* 15: 614–620.

McLellan, D.L. (1992) The feasibility of indicators and targets for rehabilitation services. *Clinical Rehabilitation,* 6: 55–66.

Malby, B. (1995) The whys and wherefores of audit, in B. Malby (ed.) *Clinical Audit for Nurses and Therapists.* London: Scutari Press.

Mansell, J. (1986) The nature of quality assurance, in J. Beswick, T. Zadik, and D. Felce (eds) *Evaluating Quality of Care.* Conference series. Kidderminster: Institute of Mental Handicap.

Mansell, J. and Beasley, F. (1990) Severe mental handicap and problem behaviour: evaluating transfer from institutions to community care, in W. Fraser (ed.) *Key Issues in Mental Retardation,* London: Routledge.

Mansell, J., McGill, P. and Emerson, E. (1994) Conceptualising service provision, in E. Emerson, J. Mansell and P. McGill (eds) *Severe Learning Disabilities and Challenging Behaviours: designing high quality services.* London: Chapman and Hall.

Marsden, J. (1993) *Outcome Funding: an innovative approach to delivering health and social care services. Report of a study tour as part of NCVO's US/UK exchange programme.* London: NCVO.

Maxwell, R.J. (1984) Quality assessment in health. *British Medical Journal,* 288: 1470–1472.

Mental Health Social Work Research and Staff Development Unit (1993) *Annual Report 1993.* Manchester: MHSWRU, University of Manchester.

Michie, S. and Kidd, J. (1994) Happy ever after. *Health Service Journal,* 3 February 1994: 27.

Miller, N. (1994) Presentation at SSRG Workshop: 'Performance Measurement in Social Services: Potential and Realities', Birmingham, 28 January 1994.

Mohide, E.A., Torrance, G.W., Streiner, D.L., Pringle, D.M. and Gilbert, R. (1988) Measuring the wellbeing of family caregivers using the time trade-off technique. *Journal of Clinical Epidemiology,* 41(5): 475–482.

Morris, J. (1993a) *Independent Lives? Community Care and Disabled People.* Basingstoke: Macmillan.

Morris, J. (1993b) The effectiveness of an Independent Living Advocate. *Social Care Research Findings,* No. 37. York: Joseph Rowntree Foundation.

Morris, J. (1994) *Your Right to Housing and Support.* London: Spinal Injuries Association.

Morris, J. (1995) *The Power to Change: commissioning Health and Social Services with disabled people.* London: Living Options Partnership, King's Fund Centre.

Morris, J. and Lindow, V. (1993) *User Participation in Community Care Services*. London: Community Care Support Force, NHS Management Executive.

Morris, L.W., Morris, R.G. and Britton, P.G. (1988a) The relationship between marital intimacy, perceived strain and depression in spouse caregivers of dementia sufferers. *British Journal of Medical Psychology*, 61: 231–236.

✹Morris, R.G., Morris, L.W. and Britton, P.G. (1988b) Factors affecting the emotional wellbeing of the caregivers of dementia sufferers. *British Journal of Psychiatry*, 153: 147–156.

Mumford, E. (1991) Need for relevance in management information systems: what the NHS can learn from industry. *British Medical Journal*, 302: 1587–1590.

Murphy, G. and Clare, I. (1991) MIETS: a service option for people with mild mental handicaps and challenging behaviour or psychiatric problems: assessment, treatment and outcomes for service users and service effectiveness. *Mental Handicap Research*, 4: 180–206.

National Association of Race Equality Advisors (1992) *Black Community Care Charter*. Birmingham: NAREA.

National Consumer Council (1987) *Performance Measurement and the Consumer*. London: NCC.

NCVO (1992) *Community Care Alliance Manifesto*. London: NCVO.

Neill, J. and Williams, J. (1992) *Leaving Hospital: elderly people and their discharge to community care*. London: HMSO.

Netten, A. (1989) *An Approach to Costing Informal Care*. Discussion Paper 637. Canterbury: PSSRU, University of Kent.

Nihira, K., Foster, R., Shellhaas, M. and Leland, H. (1974) *AAMD Adaptive Behavior Scale*. Washington DC: American Association on Mental Deficiency.

Nocon, A. (1992) *GPs' Assessments of People Aged 75 and Over*. Rotherham: Rotherham Family Health Services Authority.

Nolan, M. and Grant, G. (1992) *Regular Respite: an evaluation of a hospital rota bed scheme for elderly people*. London: Age Concern.

✴Nolan, M.R., Grant, G. and Ellis, N.C. (1990) Stress is in the eye of the beholder: reconceptualising the measurement of carer burden. *Journal of Advanced Nursing*, 15: 544–555.

North Western Regional Health Authority (1991) *Caring about Outcomes for People*. Series of Working Papers. Manchester: Community Care Services. NWRHA.

O'Boyle, C., McGee, H., Hickey, A., O'Malley, K. and Joyce, C. (1992) Individual quality of life in patients undergoing hip replacement. *Lancet*, 339, 2 May 1992: 1088–1091.

O'Brien, J. and Lyle, C. (1987) *Framework for Accomplishment*. Atlanta, Georgia: Responsive Systems Associates.

O'Driscoll, C. and Leff, J. (1993) The TAPS project. 8: design of the research study on the long-stay patients. *British Journal of Psychiatry*, 162, Supplement 19: 18–24.

Oliver, J.P.J. (1991) The social care directive: development of a quality of life profile for use in community services for the mentally ill. *Social Work and Social Services Review*, 3(1): 5–45.

Oliver, M. (1987) Re-defining disability: a challenge to research. *Research, Policy and Planning*, 5(1): 9–13.

Osborne, D. and Gaebler, T. (1992) *Reinventing Government: how the entrepreneurial spirit is transforming the public sector*. Reading, MA: Addison-Wesley.

Osborne, S.P. (1992) The quality dimension: evaluating quality of service and quality of life in human services. *British Journal of Social Work*, 22(4): 437–453.

Parker, G. (1990) *With Due Care and Attention: a review of research on informal care*, 2nd edn. London: Family Policy Studies Centre.

Parker, R., Ward, H., Jackson, S., Aldgate, J. and Wedge, P. (eds) (1991) *Looking After Children: assessing outcomes in child care*. Report of an Independent Working Party established by the Department of Health. London: HMSO.

Parker, S.G., Du, X., Striet, C., Broughton, D., Bardsley, M., Goodfellow, J. and James, O.F.W. (1994) Routine use of the Barthel Index in functional assessment of elderly hospital patients. Mimeo. Department of Medicine, University of Lancaster.

Parmenter, T.R. (1988) An analysis of the dimensions of quality of life for people with physical disabilities, in R.I. Brown (ed.) *Quality of Life for Handicapped People*. London: Croom Helm.

Pattie, A.H. and Gilleard, C.J. (1979) *Manual of the Clifton Assessment Procedures for the Elderly*. Sevenoaks: Hodder and Stoughton.

Perring, C., Twigg, J. and Atkin, K. (1990) *Families Caring for People Diagnosed as Mentally Ill: the literature re-examined*. SPRU Papers. London: HMSO.

Perry, J. and Felce, D. (1995) Objective indicators of the quality of life: how much do they agree with each other? *Journal of Community Applied and Social Psychology* 5, 1–19.

Pfeffer, N. and Coote, A. (1991) *Is Quality Good for You?* Social Policy Paper No. 5. London: Institute for Public Policy Research.

Philp, I. and Dunleavey, J. (1994) Community health assessment of elderly people. *Health and Social Care in the Community*, 2(2): 117–19.

Philp, I., Goddard, A., Connell, C., Metcalfe, A., Tse, V. and Bray, J. (1994) Development and evaluation of an information system for quality assurance. *Age and Ageing*, 23: 150–153.

Platt, S. (1985) Measuring the burden of psychiatric illness on the family: an evaluation of some rating scales. *Psychological Medicine*, 15: 383–393.

Platt, S., Weyman, A., Hirsch, S. and Hewitt, S. (1980) The Social Behaviour Assessment Schedule (SBAS): rationale, contents, scoring and reliability of a new interview schedule. *Social Psychiatry*, 15: 43–55.

Pollitt, C. (1987a) Performance measurement and the consumer: hijacking a bandwagon?, in NCC *Performance Measurement and the Consumer*. London: National Consumer Council.

Pollitt, C. (1987b) Capturing quality? The quality issues in British and American health policies. *Journal of Public Policy*, 7(1): 71–92.

Pollitt, C. (1988) Bringing consumers into performance measurement: concepts, consequences and constraints. *Policy and Politics*, 16(2): 77–87.

Pollitt, C. (1990) Performance indicators, root and branch, in M. Cave, M. Kogan and R. Smith (eds) *Output and Performance Measurement in Government: the state of the art*. London: Jessica Kingsley.

Priest, P. and McCarthy, M. (1993) Developing a measure of client needs and outcomes by a community team for people with learning disabilities. *Health and Social Care*, 1(3): 181–185.

Prosser, H. (1989) *Eliciting the Views of People with Mental Handicap: a literature review*. Manchester: Hester Adrian Research Centre, University of Manchester.

Quine, L. and Pahl, J. (1985) Examining the causes of stress in families with severely mentally handicapped children. *British Journal of Social Work*, 15: 501–517.

Quine, L. and Pahl, J. (1989) *Stress and Coping in Families Caring for a Child with Severe Mental Handicap: a longitudinal study*. University of Kent, Canterbury, Institute of Social and Applied Psychology/Centre for Health Service Studies.

Qureshi, H. (1990) *Parents Caring for Young Adults with Mental Handicap and Behaviour Problems*. Report to Department of Health. Manchester: Hester Adrian Research Centre, University of Manchester.

Qureshi, H. (1992) Young adults with learning difficulties and behaviour problems: parents' views of services in the community. *Social Work and Social Science Review*, 3(2): 104–123.

Qureshi, H. (1993) Impact on families, in C. Kiernan (ed.) *Research to Practice: learning disabilities and challenging behaviour*. Kidderminster: British Institute of Learning Disability.

Qureshi, H. (1994) The size of the problem, in E. Emerson, P. McGill and J. Mansell (eds) *Severe Learning Disabilities and Challenging Behaviours: designing high quality services*. London: Chapman and Hall.

Qureshi, H. and Walker, A. (1989) *The Caring Relationship*. Basingstoke: Macmillan.

RADAR (1993) *Disabled People Have Rights*. Interim Report. London: RADAR.

Ramsay, M., Winget, C. and Higginson, I. (1995) Review: measures to determine the outcome of community services for people with dementia. *Age and Ageing*, 24, 78–83.

Rawles, J., Light, J. and Watt, M. (1992) Quality of life in the first 100 days after suspected acute myocardial infarction – a suitable trial endpoint? *Journal of Epidemiology and Community Health*, 46: 612–616.

Raynes, N. (1986) Approaches to the measurement of care, in J. Beswick, T. Zadik and D. Felce (eds) *Evaluating Quality of Care*. Conference series. Kidderminster: British Institute of Mental Handicap.

Raynes, N. (1988) *Annotated Directory of Measures of Environmental Quality for Use in Residential Services for People with a Mental Handicap*. Manchester: Department of Social Policy and Social Work, University of Manchester.

RCP (undated) *Trials of a Set of Brief Outcome Scales to Measure the First Target of Mental Health of the Nation: report on the start-up phase*. London: Royal College of Psychiatrists Research Unit.

RCP (1995) *Health of the Nation Outcome Scales: Version 4*. London: Royal College of Psychiatrists Research Unit.

RDP (1992) Assessment and outcome indicators. Mimeo. London: Research and Development in Psychiatry.

Richardson, A., Unell, J. and Aston, B. (1989) *A New Deal for Carers*. London: King's Fund Centre.

Roberts, H., Khee, T.S. and Philp, I. (1994) Setting priorities for measurement of performance for geriatric medical services. *Age and Ageing*, 23: 154–157.

Robertson, S. (1993) *Fed and Watered: the views of older people on need, assessment and care management*. Edinburgh: Age Concern Scotland.

Rogers, A., Pilgrim, D. and Lacey, R. (1993) *Experiencing Psychiatry – Users' Views of Services*. Basingstoke: Macmillan.

Romans-Clarkson, S.E., Clarkson, J.E., Dittmer, I.D., Flett, R., Linsell, C., Mullen, P.E. and Mullin, B. (1986) Impact of a handicapped child on mental health of parents. *British Medical Journal*, 293: 1395–1397.

Royal College of Physicians (1992) *Standardised Assessment Scales for Elderly People*. London: Royal College of Physicians of London and the British Geriatrics Society.

Rutter, M., Tizard, J. and Whitmore, K. (1970) *Education, Health and Behaviour*. London: Longman.

Saunders, M.N.K., Wilson, J. and Radburn, J. (1992) Enabling consumers of social services to be heard. *Research, Policy and Planning*, 10(1): 1–5.

Schalock, R., Keith, K., Hoffman, K. and Karan, O. (1989) Quality of life: its measurement and use. *Mental Retardation* 27(1): 25–31.

Secretaries of State for Health, Social Security, Wales and Scotland (1989) *Caring for People*. Cm. 849. London: HMSO.

Shanks, J. and Gillen, V. (1992) *How Are Things? Developing Outcome Measures for Mental Health Services*. London: South East London Health Authority.

Shaw, I.F. (1984) Literature review: consumer evaluations of the personal social services. *British Journal of Social Work*, 14: 277–284.

Sheppard, M. (1991) Client satisfaction, brief intervention and interpersonal skills. *Social Work and Social Sciences Review*, 3(2): 124–149.

Shiell, A., Pettipher, C., Raynes, N. and Wright, K. (1990) Economic approaches to measuring quality of life, in S. Baldwin, C. Godfrey and C. Propper (eds) *Quality of Life: perspectives and policies*. London: Routledge.

Sigelman, C., Budd, E., Spanhel, C. and Schoenrock, C. (1981) When in doubt say 'yes': acquiescence in interviews with mentally retarded persons. *Mental Retardation*, 19, 53–58.

Sigelman, C., Budd, E., Winer, J., Schoenrock, C. and Martin, P. (1982) Evaluating alternative techniques of questioning mentally retarded persons. *American Journal of Mental Deficiency*, 85(5): 511–518.

Silburn, L. (1993) A social model in a medical world: the development of the integrated living team as part of the strategy for younger physically disabled people in North Derbyshire, in J. Swain, V. Finkelstein, S. French and M. Oliver (eds) *Disabling Barriers – Enabling Environments*. London: Sage and The Open University.

Simons, K. (1993) *Sticking Up for Yourself: self-advocacy and people with learning difficulties*. Bristol: Norah Fry Research Centre.

Simons, K. (1994) Enabling Research: people with learning difficulties. *Research, Policy and Planning*, 12(2): 4–5.

Simons, K., Booth, T. and Booth, W. (1989) Speaking out: user studies and people with learning difficulties. *Research Policy and Planning*, 7(1): 9–17.

Sinclair, I. (1990) Research and caring for people: an example of the influence of social scientists on government reports? *SRA News*, 3: 4–5.

Sinclair, I. and Clarke, R. (1981) Cross-institutional designs, in E. Goldberg and N. Connelly (eds) *Evaluative Research in Social Care*. London: Heinemann Educational.

Sinclair, I. and Williams, J. (1990) Elderly people: coping and quality of life, in

I. Sinclair, R. Parker, D. Leat and J. Williams (eds) *The Kaleidoscope of Care: a review of research on welfare provision for elderly people*. London: HMSO.

Sinclair, I., Parker, R., Leat, D. and Williams, J. (eds) (1990) *The Kaleidoscope of Care: a review of research on welfare provision for elderly people*. London: HMSO.

Slevin, M., Plant, H., Lynch, D., Drinkwater, J. and Gregory, W. (1988) Who should measure quality of life, the doctor or the patient? *British Journal of Cancer*, 57: 109–112.

Sloper, P., Glenn, S. and Cunningham, C. (1986) The effect of the intensity of training on sensory-motor development in infants with Down's syndrome. *Journal of Mental Deficiency Research*, 30: 149–162.

Sloper, P., Knussen, C., Turner, S. and Cunningham, C. (1991) Factors related to stress and satisfaction with life in families of children with Down's syndrome. *Journal of Child Psychology and Psychiatry*, 32(4): 655–676.

Smale, G., Tuson, G., Ahmad, B., Darvill, G., Domoney, L. and Sainsbury, E. (1994) *Negotiating Care in the Community*. Practice and Development Exchange, National Institute for Social Work. London: HMSO.

Smith, D. (1987) The limits of positivism in social work research. *British Journal of Social Work*, 17: 401–416.

Smith, G. (1994) Community care research: a view from the Department of Health Research and Development Division, SSI Workshop with Researchers in Community Care, February, London.

Smith, P. (1992) On the Unintended Consequences of Performance Indicator Publication. Paper presented to the 34th Annual Conference of the Operational Research Society, Birmingham, 8 September.

Smith, P. (ed.) (1996) *Outcomes in the Public Sector*. London: Taylor and Francis.

Smith, P. and Thomas, N. (1993) Contracts and Competition in Public Services. Paper presented at Association of Directors of Services, National Research Conference, Bristol, November.

Snaith, R.P., Ahmed, S.N., Mehta, S. and Hamilton, M. (1971) Assessment of the severity of primary depressive illness. *Psychological Medicine*, 1: 143–149.

Social Services Inspectorate (1989) *Homes Are For Living In*. London: HMSO.

Social Services Inspectorate (1990a) *Guidance on Standards for Residential Homes for Elderly People*. London: HMSO.

Social Services Inspectorate (1990b) *Guidance on Standards for Residential Homes for People with a Physical Disability*. London: HMSO.

Social Services Inspectorate (1990c) *Inspecting Home Care Services: a guide to the SSI method*. London: HMSO.

Social Services Inspectorate (1993) *Inspection of Assessment and Care Management Arrangements in Social Services Departments: interim overview report*. London East Inspection Group, Department of Health.

Social Services Inspectorate (1993a) *Developing Quality Standards for Home Support Services*. London: HMSO.

Social Services Inspectorate (1993b) *Inspection of Projects Funded by the Mental Illness Specific Grant*. London: HMSO.

Social Services Inspectorate/NHSE (1994) *Care Management*. London: Department of Health.

Social Services Inspectorate/NHSME (1993a) *Implementing Community Care for Younger People with Physical and Sensory Disabilities*. London: Department of Health.

Social Services Inspectorate/NHSME (1993b) *Assessment Special Study*. London: Department of Health.

Social Services Inspectorate/SWSG (1991) *Care Management and Assessment: practitioners' guide*. London: HMSO.

Social Services Research Group (1994) Performance measurement in social services: potential and realities. Workshop organized by the SSRG (Midlands Region), Birmingham, January.

Social Work Research Centre (1993) *Efficiency and Effectiveness in the Delivery of Community Care*. Research summary. Stirling: Social Work Research Centre, University of Stirling.

South East Staffordshire District Joint Planning Group (1993) Services for People with Physical/Sensory Disabilities. Discussion paper prepared by voluntary sector representatives on the South East Staffordshire District Joint Planning Group (Physical/Sensory).

Stanley, B. and Roy, A. (1988) Evaluating the quality of life of people with mental handicaps: a social validation study. *Mental Handicap Research*, 1: 197–210.

Stevens, B.C. (1972) Dependence of schizophrenic patients on elderly relatives. *Psychological Medicine*, 2: 17–32.

Stevenson, O. and Parsloe, P. (1993) *Community Care and Empowerment*. York: Joseph Rowntree Foundation.

Tanenbaum, S.J. (1994) Knowing and acting in practice: the epistemological politics of outcomes research. *Journal of Health Politics, Policy and Law*, 19(1): 27–44.

Taylor, M., Hoyes, L., Lart, R. and Means, R. (1992) *User Empowerment in Community Care: unravelling the issues*. Bristol: School for Advanced Urban Studies, University of Bristol.

Tennant, A., Geddes, J. and Chamberlain, A. (1993) Measuring rehabilitation efficiency: are we mis-using the Barthel Index? Mimeo. Rheumatology and Rehabilitation Research Unit, University of Leeds.

Thompson, C. (1995) *Research Assessment Instruments for Use with Elderly People*. Research Tools series, No. 3. London: Age Concern/Institute of Gerontology.

Todd, S., Shearn, J. and Felce, D. (1992) *The Experience and Management of Co-Residence: adults with learning difficulties living in the parental home*. Cardiff: Mental Handicap in Wales Applied Research Unit.

Todd, S., Shearn, J., Beyer, S. and Felce, D. (1993) Reflecting on change: consumers' views of the impact of the All Wales Strategy. *Mental Handicap*, 21: 128–136.

Toseland, R.W., Rossiter, C.M., Peak, T. and Smith, G.C. (1990) Comparative effectiveness of individual and group interventions to support family caregivers. *Social Work*, May: 209–217.

Townsend, J., Piper, M., Frank, A.O., Dyer, S., North, W.R.S. and Meade, T.W. (1988) Reduction in hospital readmission stay of elderly patients by a community based hospital discharge scheme: A randomised control trial. *British Medical Journal*, 297: 544–547.

Townsend, P. (1979) *Poverty in the United Kingdom*. Harmondsworth: Penguin.

Trafford SSD (1993) *Standards for Care in Residential Homes*. Sale: Trafford Borough Council.

Tunstall, J. (1966) *Old and Alone*. London: Routledge and Kegan Paul.

Twigg, J. and Atkin, K. (1994) *Carers Perceived*. Buckingham: Open University Press.

Twigg, J., Atkin, K. and Perring, C. (1990) *Carers and Services: a review of research*, SPRU Papers. London: HMSO.

UK Clearing House on Health Outcomes (1993) *Outcomes Briefing*. Introductory issue. Spring. Leeds: Nuffield Institute for Health.

Ungerson, C. (1995) Gender, cash and informal care: European perspectives and dilemmas. *Journal of Social Policy*, 24(1): 31–52.

Vetter, N.J., Jones, D.A. and Victor, C.R. (1984) Effect of health visitors working with elderly patients in general practice: a randomised control trial. *British Medical Journal*, 288: 369–372.

Victor, C.R. and Vetter, N.J. (1989) Measuring outcome after discharge from hospital for the elderly: a conceptual and empirical investigation. *Archives of Gerontology and Geriatrics*, 8: 87–94.

Walker C., Ryan T. and Walker A. (1993) *Quality of Life after Resettlement for People with Learning Disabilities*. Report to North Western Regional Health Authority. Sheffield: Department of Sociological Studies, University of Sheffield.

Walker, A. (1991) No gain without pain. *Community Care*, 18 July 1991: 14–16.

Warburton, W. (1993) Performance indicators: what was all the fuss about? *Community Care Management and Planning*, 1(4): 99–105.

Warr, B. and Kelly, D. (1992) What is meant by quality in social care?, in D. Kelly and B. Warr (eds) *Quality Counts: achieving quality in social care services*. London: Whiting and Birch Ltd.

Wattis, J.P., Butler, A., Martin, C. and Sumner, T. (1994) Outcome of admission to an acute psychiatric facility for older people: a pluralistic evaluation. *International Journal of Geriatric Psychiatry*, 9(10): 835–840.

Webb, B. and Holly, L. (1994) Evaluating a citizen advocacy scheme. *Social Care Research Findings*, No. 52. York: Joseph Rowntree Foundation.

Welsh Office (1991) *The Review of the All Wales Strategy: a view from the users*. Cardiff: Welsh Office.

Wertheimer, A. (ed.) (1991) *A Chance to Speak Out: consulting service users and carers about community care*. London: King's Fund Centre.

West Suffolk Health Authority and Suffolk County Council (1992) *A Report on Meetings Held to Obtain the Views of Older People in West Suffolk on the Provision of Services*. Ipswich: WSHASCC.

Whittaker, A., Gardner, S. and Kershaw, J. (1991) *Service Evaluation by People with Learning Difficulties*. London: King's Fund Centre.

Wilkin, D., Hallam, L. and Doggett, M. (1992) *Measures of Need and Outcome for Primary Health Care*. Oxford: Oxford University Press.

Williams, A. (1988) Applications in management, in G. Teeling Smith (ed.) *Measuring Health: a practical approach*. Chichester: Wiley.

Williams, B. (1994) Patient satisfaction: a valid concept? *Social Science and Medicine*, 38(4): 509–516.

Williams, H.S., Webb, A.Y. and Phillips, W.J. (1993) *Outcome Funding: a new approach to targeted grantmaking*, 2nd edn. Rensselaerville, New York: Rensselaerville Institute.

Williams, P. (1986) Evaluating services from the consumer's point of view, in J. Beswick, T. Zadik and D. Felce (eds) *Evaluating Quality of Care*. Conference Series. Kidderminster: British Institute of Mental Handicap.

Wilson, G. (1993) Users and providers: different perspectives on community care services. *Journal of Social Policy*, 22(4): 507–526.

Wistow, G. and Barnes, M. (1993) User involvement in community care: origins, purposes and applications. *Public Administration*, 71(3): 279–299.

Wolfe, C. (1993) List of measures used in community stroke trial. Mimeo. United Medical and Dental School, St. Thomas's Hospital, London.

World Health Organization (1980) *International Classification of Impairments, Disabilities and Handicaps*. Geneva: WHO.

Wright, K. (1987) *The Economics of Informal Care of the Elderly*. Discussion Paper 23. York: Centre for Health Economics, University of York.

Wright, K., Leedham, I. and Haycox, A. (1994) *Evaluating Community Care: services for people with learning difficulties*. Buckingham: Open University Press.

Wyngaarden, M. (1981) Interviewing mentally retarded persons; issues and strategies, in R. Bruininks, C. Meyer, B. Sigford and K. Lakin (eds) *Deinstitutionalisation and Community Adjustment of Mentally Retarded People*. Monograph No. 4. Washington DC: American Association on Mental Deficiency.

Wyn Thomas, B. (1990) *Consulting Consumers in the NHS: a guideline study. Services for Elderly People with Dementia Living at Home*. London: National Consumer Council.

Zarb, G. and Nadash, P. (1994) *Cashing in on Independence: comparing the costs and benefits of cash and services*. Belper, Derbyshire: British Council of Organisations of Disabled People.

Zarb, G., Barnes, C., Salvage, A. and Beishon, S. (1994) *Measuring Disablement in Society: outline of research project*. London: Policy Studies Institute.

Zarit, S.H., Reever, K.E. and Bach-Peterson, J. (1980) Relatives of the impaired elderly: correlates of feelings of burden. *The Gerontologist*, 20(6): 649–655.

INDEX

CHANGING SERVICES FOR OLDER PEOPLE
THE NEIGHBOURHOOD SUPPORT UNITS INNOVATION
Alan Walker and Lorna Warren

- What are the issues underpinning the trend towards innovation in the community care of older people?
- What is the nature of that innovation: how is it experienced by older people and their carers?

Changing Services for Older People sets out to address these pressing questions. It presents the findings of a major research project evaluating the outcomes of the Neighbourhood Support Units innovation in Sheffield. Key issues raised include the goals to create more flexible 'tailor made' services and the promotion of user- and carer-responsive forms of provision, shifts which are occurring in many other European countries. The aims of the book are two-fold. First, it reports on the outcomes of the initiative for older people and their carers, placing these findings in the context of current debates about community care. Second, it discusses the process of innovation in the social services, drawing on evidence gathered from policy-makers, managers and front-line workers to illustrate both the barriers to change and the ways in which successful innovation can be accomplished.

Changing Services for Older People will be invaluable to personnel in the health and social services who are considering new initiatives in service provision. It will also be a useful text for anyone wishing to gain an insight into the operation of social care services, and the experiences of older people who use those services as well as their carers.

Contents
Introduction – Changing social services in Europe – Neighbourhood support units – Older people: attitudes towards services – Older people: impact of services – The carers' perspective – Support workers – User and carer involvement in principle and practice – Conclusion – Appendix – References – Index.

208pp   0 335 19137 1 (Paperback)   0 335 19138 X (Hardback)

IMPLEMENTING THE NEW COMMUNITY CARE

Jane Lewis and Howard Glennerster

- What were the aims of the new community care policy?
- How has the policy been implemented?
- How far have the aims of the policy been achieved?

These are just some of the questions addressed by the authors of this book. They trace the implementation of the 1990 community care legislation in five local authorities between 1992 and 1994. The book suggests that central government's main aim was to bring social security spending under control. Services issues were always secondary. Nevertheless, implications both for clients and services have been important and often unintended. Local authorities have faced considerable difficulties in implementing the legislation.

The process is followed in five local authorities, one county and four London boroughs. Local authorities were faced with a mass of central government guidance and a number of key changes to make. It traces three changes in detail: the implementation of the purchaser/provider split and the creation of a social care market, the introduction of care management, and efforts to collaborate with health authorities. The book compares how the authorities tackled these issues and examines why they approached the tasks so differently. It also analyses the way in which social services departments have changed in the process and the extent to which we are seeing the end of the 'Seebohm' Departments.

Implementing the New Community Care will be of interest to students of social policy, health and social welfare and social work.

Contents
The purpose of the reforms – From high politics to local practice – Paying for community care – Changes in the structure of social services departments – Enabling authorities I: the purchaser-provider split and market information – Enabling authorities II: the market for social care – Care management I: the idea of care management – Care management II: assessing need and deciding eligibility for service – Collaboration in community care – Conclusion: what has changed? – Bibliography – Index.

240pp   0 335 19609 8 (Paperback)   0 335 19610 1 (Hardback)

'RACE' AND COMMUNITY CARE

Waqar I.U. Ahmad and Karl Atkin (eds)

This book is the first critical introduction to the area of 'race' and community care and thus fills an important gap in existing literature. The first part of the book considers the racialized constructions of community and provides a historical account of the relationship between state welfare and minority ethnic communities. Part two focuses on the nature of family obligations and the processes of social change. Part three provides case studies in 'race' and community care by focusing on disability, mental health, cash for care, and the role of the voluntary sector.

The book is essential reading for students and teachers in a broad range of courses in community care, social policy, race relations and social work. It will also be of use to practitioners, policy makers and researchers in health and social care.

Contents
'Race' and community care: an introduction – Part 1: Community, citizenship and welfare – 'Race', welfare and community care – Defining and containing diversity – Part 2: Family, obligations and community care – Family obligations and social change among Asian communities – Looking after their own? Family care-giving among Asian and Afro-Caribbean communities – Part 3: Case studies in community care – 'Yes, we mean black people too' – Representations and realities – Social security, community care – and 'race' – An opportunity for change – Bibliography – Index.

Contributors
Waqar I.U. Ahmad, Karl Atkin, Gary Craig, Charles Husband, Dhanwant K. Rai, Janet Rollings, Ossie Stuart, Charles Watters, Fiona Williams.

208pp   0 335 19462 1 (Paperback)   0 335 19463 X (Hardback)